A Recipe for C-PTSD & PNES

A True Story of Determination & Hope

DEBBIE A SAMSON

A Recipe for C-PTSD & PNES
Copyright © 2021 by Debbie A Samson

All rights reserved. No part of this publication may be reproduced, distributed, or transmitted in any form or by any means, including photocopying, recording, or other electronic or mechanical methods, without the prior written permission of the author, except in the case of brief quotations embodied in critical reviews and certain other non-commercial uses permitted by copyright law.

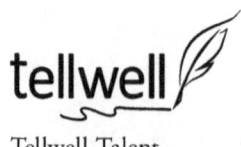

Tellwell Talent
www.tellwell.ca

ISBN
978-0-2288-5104-2 (Hardcover)
978-0-2288-5103-5 (Paperback)
978-0-2288-5105-9 (eBook)

This book is dedicated to my paternal grandmother who loved me unconditionally.

I could never have put all these memories together without the love and support of my husband, Bill; my daughter, Lisa; my son, William; and my loyal friends. Thank you. I am forever grateful.

I have written my life story truthfully. I don't want to cause unnecessary harm to individuals in my story. Without the people in my life, both the good and the not-so-good, there would be no story. It has taken me years to forgive, but I'll never forget. In forgiving, I must also look at myself and my actions in order to avoid having to ask forgiveness of myself. Therefore, I made the decision to change the names of some people in order to avoid bringing them unnecessary pain. My life has been trauma after trauma after trauma. I've made every effort possible not to bring more trauma into my life or the lives of those who are part of my story. To those who have caused me pain, I wish you no harm. Living in peace is something each of us deserves.

Cover: The picture on the cover is of the author at her childhood home when she was one year old. The teddy bear on the highchair was her favourite toy at the time. The little girl looking down on Debbie represents her identical twin sister, Daphne, who was stillborn. Debbie has felt Daphne's presence throughout her life. The photo shows how the author envisions her sister watching out for her through all of her trials in life.

Table of Contents

Foreword ix
Introduction xi

Childhood Innocence Robbed 1
A Troubled Runaway 10
Young Love 20
It Was No Honeymoon 30
Immersed in Recovery 41
Fulfilling My Calling 46
Tragedy Strikes 50
Lisa 58
William 65
Spiralling Down 75
Major Life Changes 85
An Addition to the Family 91
Complex Post-Traumatic Stress Disorder Effects 94
Psychogenic Non-Epileptic Seizures (PNES) 104
TRE® 113
Medical Cannabis 115
Lily 119
We Must Do Better for the Children 121
Life Today 123

Foreword

It is an honour to write the foreword to our mother's autobiography. We are incredibly proud of her for having the courage to write her life story. We know it was a difficult, but rewarding, undertaking. In her true style, Mom has taken the negatives in her life and turned them into positives in an effort to help others. We hope that whoever reads our mother's story will learn they can stop the trauma cycle from continuing; it can end with you.

Our mother was dealt a horrible hand, one that came with lots of loss, trauma and grief. She could have carried all of it with her and passed it on to us, but she chose to go through the agony of healing so she would not pass the poison of pain through the next generations. We are beyond grateful for the choices she made. She gave us the most amazing, memorable childhood, the kind that every kid dreams of. Having us gave Mom a chance to relive her childhood. It gave her a second chance to be a kid, with us.

Mom always had time for us; she played with us, read to us, coloured, played games, laughed with us, talked to us, listened to us. She would come into our rooms before bed and sit and talk with us about our day, sometimes for hours. She always listened, validated, supported and helped us navigate the confusing road of life. In her eyes we could do no wrong. Where other parents may have given up, she never did. Not once did she show us anything but love and support. She is our best friend.

The knowledge and information she has taught us cannot come from a book. She showed us what true love is and what it means to be family. And most importantly, she validated us. Every feeling, big or small, Mom was sure to let us know that we were heard and listened to as valuable members of our family.

We know it wasn't always easy raising the two of us, especially in our teenage years. Mom never hid her trauma from us, and she used her life lessons to help us become better, more understanding and empathic people.

We had the best fucking home on the block that all of our friends wanted to hang out at! Mom made everyone feel welcome, so much so that a lot of our friends confided in her as if she was their own mother.

Our mother is the most kind-hearted, thoughtful, supportive, caring, honest, honourable, strong woman! We are so grateful for you, Mom, and so proud of you. Through all the trauma and pain you've come out on top. Thank you for your unconditional love and acceptance. Thank you for having the courage to tell your story. Your love of helping others will endure on these pages.

Thank you, Mom, from the bottom of our hearts, for everything you've done and continue to do. Our world is a better place because of you. We are grateful for the beautiful memories you blessed us with.

We love you beyond measure. xo

Lisa Samson
William Samson

Introduction

I want to use my life story to give hope to those who suffer from mental illness, and to their loved ones who are so deeply affected by the suffering they witness; they often must stand by, feeling helpless. The stigma of mental illness, sadly, is still rampant in our society. Little by little, as each person gains the courage to speak up, we will end this stigma.

It took me a long time to let go of the shame I felt because I have a mental illness, which was intensified because I am a counsellor. I was fearful of being judged. Slowly, I gained the strength to let go of my concern about what others think of me. It is the most freeing feeling to be able to bare my soul to the world.

My dream is to have my autobiography in educational institutions around the globe. I think back to when I was in university. Had I been required to read a book such as *A Recipe for Complex PTSD & PNES*, I would have gained valuable insight into two illnesses that little is known about but so many are affected by.

Many do not understand the damage they are doing to children when they expose them to trauma and abuse. My heart breaks for the children who suffer at the hands of those who should protect them. My mental illness was preventable if the professionals I sought guidance from had been given the knowledge, and authority, to intervene. Fifty years later, children are still suffering. I hope that those who read my story who are in a position to make changes to the "system" will be inspired to take action.

Childhood Innocence Robbed

My fight for survival at birth foreshadowed my life. My identical twin sister, Daphne Pauleen, was stillborn. She took much of the nourishment and was a healthy nine-pound baby, leaving me to fight for my life. I weighed just over four pounds but, because of the malnourishment, dramatically lost weight. My grandmother often told the story of how she kept a Bible on the bottom of the stair railing, and when I turned purple and they thought I was going to die, she would get the Bible ready so she could baptize me. Babies weren't considered a Christian in the Anglican Church of the '50s until they were baptized in holy water. This has always been a sore point for me. How dare they bury my perfectly healthy, beautiful baby sister in an unmarked grave in some corner of the cemetery just because she wasn't a "Christian"? *I'll fix that*, I thought to myself when I learned of this atrocity.

I was born Deborah Ann (after Debbie Reynolds, my father's favourite actress) on August 25, 1958, at the James Paton Memorial Hospital in Gander, Newfoundland. My parents wanted to name me Debbie but it wasn't a so-called "Christian" name, so the Anglican minister refused. Although I wasn't christened Debbie, I've always been known as Debbie.

As I reflect on my childhood, it's difficult to find happy moments. I lived with my father (Jim), mother (Ruby), brother (David) and paternal grandmother. I no longer refer to Jim and Ruby as "Mom" and "Dad" because one has to earn—and deserve—those titles. Jim and Ruby lost the right many years ago. For a long time, I secretly wished I was adopted and that one day my adoptive parents would come looking for me.

I grew up in Burnside, Newfoundland, a small, rural community where "things" were kept hush. At a very young age I realized that in order to survive the abuse that was happening at our house, I had to make every effort to become invisible. I no longer call it a home because a home constitutes happiness, love and belonging, none of which I felt. When I visited friends' homes for birthday parties I felt an incredible warmth and love that was missing from our house.

My one saving grace was Nannie, who took me under her wing and became my protector. In her eyes, Debbie could do no wrong. She was my world and the one person who taught and showed me unconditional love. If not for her, I would likely not be alive to tell this story. She showed me how to survive—and even shine—in an environment no child should ever have to endure. Despite being a victim of her own son's abuse, she never turned her back on me, always doing her best to shelter me from the storms which overtook our dwelling. Having lost her husband just a few years prior to my birth, my arrival gave her a sense of purpose. As Maya Angelou said, "People will forget what you said, people will forget what you did, but people will never forget how you made them feel." When I read her words I'm reminded of my beautiful grandmother; she made me feel like the most special girl in the world.

In reality, Nannie and I needed each other. She had completely lost the sight in one eye and saw only shadows in the other eye due to cataracts. The doctor could not guarantee she would not completely lose the little sight she had, so she chose to not have them removed. She was a strong, independent woman who refused to give in. A representative from the Canadian National Institute for the Blind (CNIB) came to visit Nannie and gave her a white cane. However, she staunchly refused to use that cane. Instead, I became her guide, helping her manoeuvre her way to visit her friends' houses, the grocery store and to church on the gravel roads in our community.

Whenever I hear old church hymns, I sit and soak up the memory of Nannie's soft, angelic voice as she sang from her hymn book with the enlarged print (even though she didn't need the book, as she had memorized the words of those treasured hymns). "How Great Thou Art" is particularly special to me. The lyrics and my memory of Nannie singing it bring me a heavenly feeling of comfort and peace. When I hear it, my body sinks into a deep, relaxed state. I'm so thankful Nannie instilled in me a belief of something greater than us. It has helped my spirituality grow and brought me peace when I felt I had nowhere else to turn.

I cherish those memories, particularly the ones where we would sit with her elderly friends having lunch while they chatted and reminisced. One home particularly intrigued me because they had a hatch in the kitchen. Someone would always lift the hatch, climb down the ladder and bring up goodies for our lunch. I looked forward to the chewy candies and delicious fruit cake.

Nannie had total faith and trust in me, especially as I got older. She didn't believe in keeping her money in a bank, so she kept it in a small box in a trunk in her bedroom. Occasionally, she would ask me to count her money as she didn't trust my father, mother and brother (rightly so). Although her vision was poor, she always knew exactly how much money was there, and I felt very proud to know that she trusted me with her life savings.

I enjoyed spending time with my grandmother. The memories I have of us are quite special. At that time, horses and sheep roamed freely around the community, so one of our rituals was to gather horse manure in a bucket to spread around her beautiful rose trees for fertilizer. Nannie loved her trees and flower beds. To this day, I cannot pass a rose tree without smelling a rose and absorbing the memory it evokes of my amazing grandmother.

Despite Nannie's best efforts to protect me, it was impossible to eliminate the effects that an abusive, alcoholic, narcissist father had on a vulnerable child. The physical scars he inflicted pale in comparison to the emotional and verbal ones.

I attended a small two-room school in Burnside from Grade 1 to Grade 4. I was an A student and loved going to school. My Grade 3 report card says, "Debbie is an excellent pupil." Not only was learning a pleasure for me, but it was also an escape from the realities of living in an abusive home.

I dreaded coming home after school or when I had been outside playing because I never knew what was in store. What kind of a mood would he be in? Would he be drunk? Would he lash out at me, as was commonplace, for no apparent reason or for something he imagined I had done wrong? It could be an all-out fight with Ruby over something as trivial as not cooking his meal the way he expected. Would I have to listen to his never-ending speeches about his greatness or how important he thought himself to be? I dreaded these speeches. I was forced to sit at the kitchen table for what seemed liked hours, listening to him rant about his talents that no one else possessed, his admiration of himself, his exaggerations, and on and on and on. I dared not look away or show a lack of interest as that would be grounds to be terrorized, which took many forms; he had to emphasize his control and superiority over me.

Throughout my life I've tried hard to turn the negatives into positives, as I believe that if we look hard enough we will find gratitude, even in hardships. These speeches taught me how to be an excellent listener, and this skill came naturally to me as I went on to become a counsellor. I often think of the CBC movie *Jack*, about the late Jack Layton. Jack's mother-in-law, Ho Sze, says, "Every disappointment is a gift. We just have to unwrap it." I've strived to live my life by unwrapping my many disappointments, and I've learned to turn them into gifts. Many of my "gifts" have given me the ability to help others, which is my ultimate goal for writing my autobiography.

Jim lacked empathy and delighted in seeing others suffer. His abuse was sometimes subtle. One excruciating example was when he made a fist and scrubbed his knuckles over my head; it hurt so badly but I was not permitted to show any pain, tears or feelings as this would set him off and he would scrub harder. He took great pleasure in making me bow down to him, sometimes in the form of tickling, but his tickling was with his long fingernails that scraped my skin. The more I told him to stop the more he hurt me. During these occasions Nannie would intervene but she was putting herself at risk, as he would oftentimes turn his anger toward her. She saved me from as much as she could.

Like many things in life which are learned in childhood, one has to strive to unlearn unhealthy behaviours. Being overwhelmed with worry was something I learned very early. I spent countless hours sitting with my grandmother at the foot of her bed, watching out the window into the dark night sky where there were rarely any lights. We would watch for the lights of Jim's car as he drove the six miles from the nearest bar. I became anxious, wondering if he would make it home safe and alive. The added worry was wondering what kind of mood he would be in. Fear gripped my grandmother and I as we watched and waited to see the lights of his vehicle.

Most nights he staggered in and all hell would break loose. He was always angry about an event that had happened while he was at the bar or an imaginary event he thought happened to my grandmother, mother, brother or myself. He would yell, curse and break things. I would stay in my bedroom, pretending I was asleep and praying that he wouldn't come upstairs and take his anger out on me, but I couldn't sleep; I was terrified. I would lie in my bed, crying and praying for peace. The fear that overtook my mind and my body is a fear that now, in my '60s, I can still feel. Even as I write these words today, my body feels the same fear.

One night that will haunt me until I die is when he fired a gun at Ruby as she ran out of the house. She could not please him, no matter how hard she tried. He always found something to fight with her about. That night, he falsely accused her of having an affair with a man in our community and was adamant that David was fathered by this man, not him. This was the furthest thing from the truth but it just shows the kind of man he was.

Jim would make it home after his days, which would run into evenings, of drinking but I cannot imagine how he safely got home without killing himself or someone else. I dragged him out of his vehicle on a number of occasions because he had passed out over the steering wheel or was hanging out the door. I would beg and plead with him to wake up and come in the house. He couldn't stand up, let alone talk, without slurred speech. These episodes pre-empted my childhood and forced me to grow up too fast.

Burnside is an eighteen-kilometre boat ride to the island of St. Brendan's, and a ferry makes the run on a regular basis. However, when residents of the island needed transportation outside of the normal ferry schedule they often called on Jim to transport them in his motor boat. A lot of heavy drinking went on during some of those trips. Jim would leave the house, sometimes when the weather was not safe for such travel. Other times he would take the boat out on the water when he was under the influence and should not have been doing so.

Jim was a daredevil who had nine lives. During one of his adventures on the water he was unable to bring his boat back to Burnside because a storm rolled in. He made it safely to an island, but no one knew if he was dead or alive or where he was. Search and Rescue were called and, as soon as the weather cleared, a chopper began the search for him. Ruby and Nannie were very worried and hardly able to contain their fear, which was transferred to this little girl who went to her room and prayed that Jim would be found safe and alive. When he came home he was angry that

Search and Rescue had been called and made it clear that he was just fine and didn't need to be rescued.

Jim not only took chances with his own life but he was reckless with others' lives as well, which I realized at a very young age. I didn't want to go anywhere with him. There were occasions where he forced me to go, despite my insistence, as well as Nannie's, that I wanted to stay home. One such occasion was a trip in his boat to visit St. Brendan's. On the way back to Burnside a vicious wind and rain storm blew in. David, Ruby and I were terrified. I can still picture the bow of the boat going under the water as each wave came crashing against the boat. In an effort to alleviate our fear, David and I made a game of watching the waves hit. It is a trip I will never forget and one that probably started my fear of boats. Nannie was home worried sick, fearing that she would never see us again. When we arrived home safely, Jim, although he rarely acknowledged fear, admitted that he was worried.

I liked to spend time with Nannie when I was little. Jim, Ruby and David often went to visit Jim's friends and their families where a bunch of men would sit around drinking, arguing and swearing. I despised these outings. Nannie was usually able to make a case for me staying home with her, which I was very grateful for. However, there were occasions where Jim forced me to go with them. One Sunday afternoon, I was forced to accompany them to a gathering at a popular beach just off the highway to Eastport. There were no girls; just boys for David to play with. I felt very out of place. Jim was drinking, and I was terrified on the ride back to Burnside because he was swerving all over the road and almost went in the ditch a few times. Trips like this were the norm, and they instilled a fear of driving in me that has taken many years to overcome.

When an individual was picked up for impaired driving in the 1960s the police took the license plates off of their vehicle. I vividly remember the day they showed up to take the plates off Jim's car. Nannie and I were watching out the kitchen window. She was angry and embarrassed that this was happening.

I am four years older than David. My earliest memory of him was a turbulent flight he, Ruby and I took from Newfoundland to Nova Scotia when he was an infant. A man seemed to try and console Ruby who was very fearful, and this fear was projected on me at that young age. I suffer from a fear of flying to this day. I was a little too young to understand what was happening, but I believe Ruby may have been attempting to leave Jim. Throughout my childhood I always hoped she would leave him. Without Jim in the picture, Ruby could have been a good parent. However, his control over her left her powerless.

A memory that has always stuck with me was that of a toy wash tub and scrubbing board that was given to me, probably as a Christmas gift. In the early 1960s we did not have a washing machine so Ruby and Nannie washed clothes on a scrubbing board, in a large, galvanized wash tub. I distinctly remember wanting to wash my doll's clothes with my toy tub and scrubbing board but was broken hearted because Ruby would not allow me to. These types of incidents were common…what other children were permitted to do, I was not.

I was chastised for leaving my doll's carriage beside the house when Jim was shingling the roof. I was a little girl trying to play as children should without having to be on guard. Nannie stepped in to save me from Jim's relentless yelling and cursing. The carriage now had a hole in it where a shingle fell from the roof and went through the hood. Each time I played with that carriage I saw the tape that was put on the hole. It was always a reminder to try harder to be perfect. And I wonder why I became a perfectionist!

One time, a cousin a few years older than me came to visit with her family. This was their first and only visit. She was wearing a pretty sweater and, of course, wanting to be like her, I went to my room and put on my sweater. Jim was outraged; screaming and yelling, he sent me back to my room and made me take off the sweater. Nannie was mortified; her and I were embarrassed. There was absolutely no reason for his behaviour other than to show that he was in control. We had few relatives in Newfoundland, and my grandmother, being one who loved to have company, was very saddened after this incident. She never saw her sister-in-law again.

My memories of Christmas as a child are bittersweet. Jim was the one who woke David and I up to see what Santa had brought. Opening the gifts—one from Santa, and the others from family—was a happy occasion. But once the gifts were open, it was just another day where we walked on eggshells, not knowing what to expect from Jim's Jekyll and

Hyde personality. The happiness of that hour on Christmas morning is overshadowed by memories of the fear I felt. Memories of moonshine and beer being brewed, of Jim being in a drunken stupor, of men coming to the house to drink. Memories of the arguing, yelling, fighting and the dread I felt knowing that Christmas was a time of uncertainty and abuse. My childhood Christmas memories have left me with intense sadness around this time of year as an adult. While I watch others who are happy and jovial in the spirit of Christmas, I just want to retreat in a corner until it's all over and the memories fade again for another year.

My godmother and godfather lived just up the road from our house, and I would visit with them as often as possible when I was little. There was an implied rule that we were not permitted to talk about what happened at home, and I secretly wished someone would take me away from the place which was supposed to be "home," to a place where I could feel like I belonged. At a young age, I thought people in our community didn't know what was "secretly" happening behind the four walls of our house. It was only when I visited my godparents' daughter a few years ago that I learned people did know what we endured in that house. My godparents' daughter told me that when I left their house my godmother would say, "I wonder what poor little Debbie is going back home to." These words brought much needed comfort and validation.

There was, in my opinion, a prelude to the mental illnesses I would develop later in life. I fell over a cliff by the ocean in front of our house in Burnside when I was six or seven. I have no recollection of falling or what preceded it. This was the beginning of a mysterious medical condition that was followed by numerous trips to the Janeway Children's Hospital in St. John's where I had a number of EEGs. Jim and Ruby were informed that I was experiencing convulsions, with no known cause. A couple of years later I experienced a second convulsion. This one was in my sleep. I wet my bed while sleeping with my grandmother. I was not a bedwetter so my grandmother immediately became concerned.

My first memory of this convulsion was sitting on the daybed in the kitchen while Jim showed me pages in the Eaton's catalogue. He pointed out an iron and asked me what it was.

"That's an iron," I said.

The relief on Nannie's face is etched in my mind. Until that point, I was unaware of my surroundings and unable to respond. I believe these mysterious incidents were a result of the stress under which I was forced to live as a child. It was my body's way of trying to release the flight/flight/freeze responses that had accumulated in my nervous system.

I first faced living without Nannie when I was ten years old. Jim accepted a job in St. John's where the family moved, but Nannie stayed in Burnside. It was a whole new world for me. I missed Nannie and the comfort she brought me. She was no longer there to protect me from the ravages of child abuse.

Ruby suffered from depression and often wasn't present for me, so Nannie filled the mother role in my life. I've come to realize that Ruby didn't bond with me as a mother typically does. During the period we lived in St. John's, Ruby suffered a major depressive episode. She was hospitalized for an extended period where she underwent shock treatment. She had lived with clinical depression all her life and, undoubtedly, the abuse she endured from Jim exacerbated the illness. I believe she was doing her best to fight it on her own, but it all came to a head when she charged at me with a kitchen knife. I was able to escape from her long enough to call Jim who immediately came home. David and I then had a babysitter stay with us while Jim worked, until Rudy was well enough to return home. As an adult who knows depression both personally and professionally, I now understand what was happening to Ruby. As a ten-year-old child, however, being around her was terrifying. The rage in her eyes as she charged at me with the knife is a vision still very vivid in my mind.

A Troubled Runaway

When Jim was laid off from his job in St. John's he decided to move to London, Ontario, where Ruby's father had gotten him a job with the Ford Assembly Plant. A kid from rural Newfoundland did not fit in with other children in this city, so I was an eleven-year-old fish out of water. I soon understood what it meant to be bullied, even by Ruby's brothers, who were a few years older than me. My "Newfie" accent was their prime target. The fact that I was a "goody-goody" seemed to bring them delight as they subtly demeaned me.

We lived in a ground floor apartment that had a fenced-in swimming pool beside the building. That's where I learned to either swim or drown when Larry, my uncle who was merely three years my senior, pushed me into the pool. I struggled to keep my head above the water, flinging my arms wildly and gasping for air while stretching to reach the side of the pool. Larry watched on, not realizing that I couldn't swim. The fighter in me instinctively took over, as I battled for my life. I wanted to cry for help, but I couldn't get enough air into my lungs to scream, and we were alone in the fenced-in, unguarded pool. As I kicked and clawed desperately at the water, I got closer to the side of the pool where I reached out and clung to the edge. In my counsellor training, I learned that a near-drowning is one of life's most traumatic experiences.

I was a good kid who was eager to make friends when I started school in London. Leba, a Jewish girl, reached out to me on the first day in my new school, and we clicked right away. I asked if I could bring her home, but, to my dismay, Jim was adamant that I was not to hang around with her because she was Jewish. He was prejudice for no reason other than the fact that she was Jewish. I was heartbroken and lonely. As I reflect on the fact that Jim would not allow me to be friends with Leba, I've concluded that I could have avoided the trouble and trauma if Jim was even a little less narcissistic. I was a good kid who never got into trouble, as was Leba. I was desperate for a place to belong, and Leba provided that for me; I know we could have been good friends. Because of Jim's prejudice and need to control, I was forced to look elsewhere for friends and acceptance.

A "goody-goody" Newfie was not cool in the popular clique in London. To fit in, I had to conform to lower standards in order to find belonging and acceptance. I found a place to belong in a group of kids who were the badasses. They smoked, drank, did drugs and had no rules at home. This is where I began to experiment. By age twelve I was addicted to cigarettes. I experimented with alcohol, LSD, hash and sniffing solvents.

During one episode while I was stoned on LSD, I had to go home for supper. I sat at the table watching Jim eat a hamburger as if he was in a slow-motion film. It was hilarious and I couldn't stop giggling. Naturally, he was furious with me. I hurriedly ate my supper and escaped to the living room where a movie was on TV. In my stoned state it appeared in slow motion. I still smile to myself when I think about it because it really was funny. But not all of my LSD trips were as pleasant as this particular one. Some caused paranoia and unpleasant hallucinations. Another gave me the sensation that my body was light, like a feather, which tempted me to fly off a high-rise balcony. Thankfully, friends intervened and I lived to tell the story.

I strived to keep my friends a secret from Jim because I knew he would not approve. He was very strict and controlling, whereas my newfound friends had no rules. There were places I was not permitted to go. Of course, I lied about my whereabouts and was vigilant when it came to my curfew.

Because my uncles were only a few years older than me, they were aware of my new friends, what we were doing and where we were going. One evening I received a phone call from a guy who told me where I had been the prior evening and who I was with. He hung up while I sat in shock and disbelief. Jim was within earshot and, although I was scared of his reaction, I was more fearful of this unknown guy. Jim called the police, and I was instructed to keep the person on the phone if another call came in, and to immediately press a series of numbers which would trace the call. The police traced the next call to a gas station where Ben, my uncle who was six years older than me, worked. When confronted, he denied making the calls and was adamant that he had no knowledge of who did. There were no further calls.

The prank calls opened a rift between Jim, and Ruby's family. They also made life harder for me, as Jim had learned the truth about who I was hanging around with and where I was. I was grounded, which made it even more difficult to live in this family. I had no escape. I was trapped again and had no choice but to abide by his rules. After what seemed like forever, Jim agreed to allow me to go out but with very strict rules and a nine o'clock curfew. There was a large clock in the entrance way of the apartment. According to my watch I was on time, but the entranceway clock said it was 9:03. There he stood, his eyes wild with rage, shouting at me because I was late. I attempted to defend myself but it fell on deaf ears. He grabbed his shoe and hit me across the back and, seeing this didn't cause enough pain, he hit me across the back with his hand. I wore his handprint for days. I was then sent to my room, grounded again.

I had reached a point in my life where I was no longer the "goody-goody." I had become a badass like my friends and the warrior in me began to rebel. Nannie and I shared a bedroom on the ground floor apartment. I slit the screen in the window with a razor blade, heart racing, fearing Jim would catch me before I escaped. I jumped out of the window. When my feet landed on the ground I ran as fast as my legs could carry me until I knew I was far enough away that he couldn't see me. My friends, of course, were still out and I quickly caught up with them and was welcomed to a place I felt I belonged and was accepted. It wasn't long before a police car drove up to a field where I was hanging out with my friends. Jim stepped out of the patrol car along with an officer. His words still echo in my mind:

"You take her, we don't want her; she's trouble."

With that, I was off for processing with the Children's Aid Society (CAS). It shocked me that my own father could just give me away but, on the other hand, I was relieved that I didn't have to go back where he was. I had grown to dislike and fear him.

My first placement with CAS was at May Court House, which was a receiving home that housed children of all ages. They ranged from extremely troubled to completely innocent. Some were there because their behaviour was out of control, like mine, and others because of their parents'/guardians' issues.

I remained defiant at May Court House. I observed the behaviour of the older children and knew I had to emulate them in order to survive and fit in. Witnessing aggression from the older residents taught me that I had to follow their lead to gain their acceptance. There were rules, chores and responsibilities at May Court House. I soon learned that those who disregarded the rules were the ones who won respect from the other children. I craved to be one of those children and so I disobeyed and acted out.

During one episode in which I became verbally and physically violent toward the staff, I was locked in a padded room (secure isolation) for what felt like an eternity. There were no windows. There was nothing in the room. The door, with no windows, was locked. I could not escape! This is my first recollection of having claustrophobia and a panic attack. How could someone do this to a twelve-year-old child! Thankfully, these rooms are no longer used by CAS.

What I've written thus far has flowed well and not caused emotional side effects. That is, until I wrote about the padded room—an event I had not yet processed. As I wrote I became angry, could feel it wanting to explode in me. The fighter in me came out and, not sure where I would go with it, I called CAS in London, Ontario. I explained what I was writing and was relieved to hear they no longer use padded rooms. With that, my emotions turned to sadness and I cried on the phone with the lady from CAS, who was understanding and compassionate. I called my daughter, Lisa, who is always there for me, to let it out. Her and I had a productive chat and, as always, she encouraged me to "feel," and she spoke the validating words I needed to hear. I later had an appointment with my counsellor, which gave me another opportunity to process the event.

After May Court House, I was placed in a foster home for about three hours. A social worker took me to the home, introduced me to the foster parents, escorted me to my bedroom and left me there while she went to talk to them. The foster father soon appeared in my bedroom, and I instinctively knew he wasn't there to welcome me. I don't remember his exact words but I do remember the sick and disgusting feeling in my stomach after he rubbed his body against me and touched my breasts. I loudly cursed him out, ran downstairs and screamed to the social worker that I was not staying in a house with this pervert. I was whisked out of there immediately. I contacted CAS in 1984, 1992 and 1994 to ask for information regarding my placements. Interestingly, the foster home with the pervert is not listed.

My next placement was at Dixon Receiving Home, a family home on a farm in a rural area. It was isolated, with no others houses in sight. This family had other foster children in addition to their own. They were a loving, caring family and, had I been in a different mindset, it would have been an ideal placement for me. However, I stayed only a week and rebelled against every effort they made to love me. I refused to eat their meals, lashed out whenever they tried to include me in family activities and fought with the other children. Deep down, a part of me did not want to behave this way but the dominant part of me was angry. I had nowhere to express the anger other than at the people who were trying to help me.

My social worker, an amazing woman who treated me like her own, came to talk to me. I threw a tantrum and slapped her in the face. I was a child in need of help but, in the '70s, there was no help. I didn't receive the counselling I so desperately needed. Throughout my life I often thought of this caring social worker. After an exhaustive search, I found her in 2012, and we communicated back and forth. Here is an excerpt from an email I sent to her:

"I have never forgotten the kindness you showed me, and I wanted to thank you for being one of very few people in my childhood who showed unconditional love to me. I remember not being very kind in return and deep down in my heart I wanted to but the rebellious child wouldn't allow me. I was so confused at that time. It was a difficult childhood and it took me a long time to figure it all out. I eventually learned that I wasn't the 'bad' girl; I was the girl who was reacting to the abuse she was enduring. I remember you gave me a necklace and card when we left Ontario for Newfoundland, and I cherished it and was very disappointed to discover that it went missing after I left home.

Thank you, Anne, from the bottom of my heart for all you tried to do for a girl who was so confused. I am sure many other children in my situation also benefitted from the love, caring and kind-heartedness you showed to them, as you did to me."

After Dixon Receiving Home I was again placed at May Court House, until a room became available at Dufferin Street Group Home. Rick and Pauleen, the group home parents, were a loving, gentle and supportive couple. I was assigned a new social worker, Freda, whom I did not get along with at all. The first several months at the group home were uneventful, and I actually felt comfortable and fit in well with the girls and the routine.

The girls at the group home shared a room. When Susan moved there she was assigned a room with me, which is when things went downhill. The already vulnerable child I was didn't need much encouragement to take the wrong path. Susan and I hung out at a drop-in centre for young people that was just down the street from the group home. Eventually we became involved with young men who were much older. Susan was fourteen and I was thirteen, although we looked older and lied about our age. We dressed provocatively and wore a lot of make-up. At the time, Alice Cooper was popular and we often did our make-up like him, with multiple black lines coming off of our eyes.

We routinely missed curfew, skipped school, and we eventually ran away. We panhandled for money on the streets and stole what we needed to in order to survive. Our bed was wherever we ended up for the night. Oftentimes we put ourselves in extremely dangerous situations. We stayed low key as we didn't want to be found and taken back to the care of CAS. One of our temporary residences was with a man in his 50s. He treated us well and even fed us and permitted us to use his apartment to party. The first time I got drunk was at his place. I had consumed an excessive amount of wine. I recall getting the spins, laying on the cold bathroom floor, vomiting profusely. I soon realized he wasn't allowing us to stay there out of the goodness of his heart. He wanted something in return, which I abruptly found out one day when I entered the kitchen. He grabbed me and pushed me to the floor. He held me down while he undid his pants and pushed my face toward his penis. I was scared, in shock and disgusted. I fought him and, to this day, I don't know how I managed to get away from his grip and escape.

We had gotten to know members of motorcycle gangs in London, and we hung out at their club. Although I spent a lot of time with these men, deep down I was not comfortable, as I knew what they were capable of doing to me. One of the bikers, an older guy named Ray, was my guardian angel. We had been partying with some of the bikers when I was forced into a bedroom. Although I was promiscuous, I was not at all interested in sexual activity with any of them. The fighter in me kicked in, and I screamed and yelled. Suddenly he grabbed a gun from the night table. I froze! Terror gripped every inch of my body as I sank back on the bed. Suddenly, the door flew open and Ray charged into the room. He grabbed the other biker by the shirt, lifting him from the bed, and made it clear that he was to leave me alone. Ray commanded respect from the other bikers, and I am forever indebted to my guardian angel who intervened and saved me from an assault or even worse.

That night Susan and I stayed at Ray's place where it felt safe. I couldn't remember the last proper meal we had, so we were hungry in the morning. I can honestly say that I know what it feels like to be hungry—really hungry! We searched the cupboards and came up with only a box of macaroni and a can of tomato soup. Neither of us knew how to cook macaroni, but we had heard that if you threw it at the wall and it stuck there, it was cooked. That macaroni/tomato soup mixture was like eating a meal fit for a princess. It was delicious. It felt so good to get food into a very empty belly. The taste of satisfying real hunger is one that will stay with me for as long as I live.

With no roof over our heads or food to eat, Susan and I decided to return to the group home. Naturally, there were consequences for our actions. Within a matter of days, Susan and I decided we couldn't stand the confinement and, once again, we were on the run. We knew the authorities would be looking for us, so in an effort to disguise ourselves, we went to a public washroom and dyed our hair. We had to run out of that washroom as a cleaner came in and caught us. It was a mad dash out of one mall, across the street, with hair dye dripping and people staring. We made it to another public washroom where we finished dying our hair. I transformed my dark brown hair to strawberry blonde.

We hitchhiked from London, Ontario, to Montreal, Quebec, a distance of over seven hundred kilometres. We hitched rides with truckers and, fortunately, the trip was uneventful. Upon arriving in Montreal, we sought out a nightclub. I was surprised to find the waitresses serving drinks, along with pills, on trays. Within minutes Susan and I were picked up by a couple of guys dressed in leather who I assumed belonged to a biker gang.

Johnny, with his dark brown, shoulder-length hair, was an attractive man. When I looked into his dark eyes and listened to his deep voice I became weak at the knees; I was drawn to him. He took a liking to me and it was obvious that he wanted me as his "old lady." It didn't take long to realize that Johnny was not the charming man I was falling for; he turned out to be the devil in disguise.

Susan and I accompanied Johnny and his friend to an apartment. They were both tough-looking, rough-talking guys who made me nervous. I was forced to sleep in Johnny's room, and he wanted sex. While he repeatedly tried to push himself on me, I lied to him and said I had VD. I begged him to stop. He became agitated, pushed me in the bed and told me to stay there, that he wasn't finished with me. I was petrified with fear, as it was obvious that he was extremely irritated with me. Luckily for me, he had consumed an excessive amount of alcohol and drugs. Within no time he had fallen asleep. I had not overlooked the fact that there was a handgun beside his pillow.

I silently, carefully edged my body to the side of the bed, as far away from him as possible. Meanwhile, I was fighting the panic rising. I trembled inside, hardly daring to breath. My heart pounded. My thoughts raced. Who would save me? There was no one! Where was Susan? I had to escape! I didn't want to die! What if he woke up? How could I get out of this place in the dark?

I lay there for what seemed like hours, not moving a muscle. He began snoring, and I waited until it intensified to take my chance. I slowly and cautiously put my feet on the cold floor and slipped into my shoes. My legs felt like jelly, as my heart pounded in my chest while creeping across the darkened room and out the door.

To my surprise and relief, Susan, who had also escaped, was waiting for me outside the door. Our timing was perfect. We quickly and quietly tiptoed out of the apartment. Upon reaching the street we ran as fast as we could until we felt we were safely away from the dangers that had gripped us.

Until I started writing about the incident at Johnny's, I didn't realize I hadn't processed the trauma I experienced. I had stuffed my feelings far down and built a wall on top of them. As I wrote, all the unprocessed trauma in my body began to swell and broke through the wall. It became overwhelming. I went into panic mode, anxiety increasing, until I started to sob and shake. My body froze. My mind went blank. I was alone in the house.

Instinctively I knew I needed someone to talk me through this horror. I reached for the phone and pressed the caller list. Thank goodness Lisa's number appeared. Through my sobs, I briefly explained what had just happened. Her gentle voice and words slowly brought me out of my terror.

"Mom, press Save," she said.

I followed her instructions.

"Now, close your laptop."

Again, I complied. While taking deep breaths I listened carefully as Lisa guided me through a technique I had taught her. I imagined putting the whole ordeal into a box and shipping it away in a truck. This was incredibly helpful. Lisa then wanted to know what my immediate plans were. Coincidently, my friend Line and I had planned a walk in the woods within the next half hour. I focused on getting ready. After the relaxing walk and a chat with Line, I was back to my old self. I felt lighter.

For the next few days we wandered the streets, panhandling for money, eating where we could and sleeping in inconspicuous places. Without any consideration for our safety, Susan and I decided to hitchhike just to get a change of scenery. Three guys in a car picked us up and proceeded to an isolated gravel pit. There they threatened us with a crowbar while they raped us. Before they forced us out of the car, one of them got out. When they released us, my first thought was to get the license plate number as they drove away. However, the one who had gotten out was smart enough to put tree branches in the openings around the plate so the number wasn't visible. Despite the ordeal we had just been through, I became angry as I knew we would not be able to get justice for their heinous crime.

Susan and I walked and walked, having no idea where we were. Eventually we flagged down a police officer and disclosed what had just taken place. We were taken to the detachment. They soon learned we were runaways from CAS in London. We described the guys in the car and pleaded that they find them, but the police didn't take us seriously. We were searched and put in a jail cell! Talk about adding insult to injury. I will never forget the night I spent in a jail cell! One has to be heartless to put a thirteen-year-old girl who has just been raped in a jail cell!

The following morning, we were put on a flight to London. Susan and I went our separate ways, and I didn't see her again.

I told the social worker about our ordeal, but the only help I received from CAS was a doctor's appointment for a physical examination. No further action was taken by CAS regarding the rape in Montreal. Again, not being taken seriously was upsetting. I contacted CAS in 1994 regarding my concerns. In a letter from their Intake and Child Abuse Services Director I was informed that their files "make no reference to any alleged rape by three men while Deborah was on the run in Montreal." I was naïve to expect anything different.

After the "run" to Montreal, CAS placed me in a juvenile detention home, a locked facility in which my every move was monitored. Essentially, I was in a prison for teens. I was very unhappy, felt trapped and saw no way out of my misery. The one saving grace in the detention home was school which, of course, was mandatory to attend. I hadn't attended school while living on the streets and on the run. Although I missed a lot of the curriculum, I was determined to study hard and succeed, and I did. One of my progress reports from London Public Schools states, "Debbie finds 'failure' in any respect very difficult to accept and works hard to overcome it. Perhaps it would be beneficial to her to learn to laugh at her mistakes." Mrs. Morrison had great insight into my personality. She summed up my drive to succeed in everything I have taken on in my life.

Coincidentally, Jim had injured his back and was no longer able to work. He had contacted CAS, as they were returning to Newfoundland. Subsequently, we attended family counselling. In those sessions I had the opportunity to voice my concerns about the environment at home. I felt the sessions went well, as Jim and Ruby actually listened. We came to an agreement which sounded reasonable, and I was hopeful that things had changed.

The whole family drove back to Newfoundland in the summer of 1972. What stood out for me on that long drive was the feeling of being trapped. I had changed. I had been forced to grow up too fast. At the tender ages of twelve and thirteen I had faced horrendous situations that no human should ever have to endure.

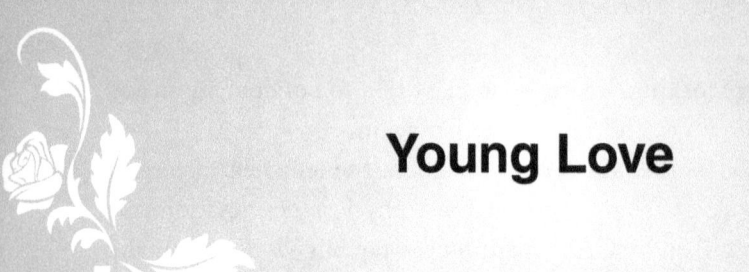

Young Love

Nothing changed when I moved back with Jim and Ruby.

"I straightened you out," he said to me.

If people in the small community of Burnside didn't know what was happening behind the walls of our house when I was a little girl, they would soon learn about it. I became reacquainted with my childhood friends, who were intrigued when I told them some of my experiences. I had given myself a small heart tattoo on my pinkie finger when I was living on the streets, and my friends were amazed; they had never seen a tattoo on a young girl.

Burnside changed while we were living in Ontario. During my absence the small, two room school had closed. The children were now being bused to a larger school, eight kilometres away, in Eastport. This was going to be a new adventure for me, and I was about to be introduced to a whole new group of friends. We moved during the summer so we had plenty of time to just hang out. It meant trying to find rides to Eastport but there was usually a parent who was going that way.

One afternoon Jim and Ruby had driven my friend, Lynda, and I to Eastport where they dropped us off at the local hangout. As we were exiting the car I jokingly, but with embarrassment, told Ruby to duck out of sight so no one would see her with rollers in her hair. I thought no more about it, but I found out later that Jim was enraged.

I returned home with Lynda, which was rare. I didn't bring friends home because either Jim would disapprove of them or I was afraid of violence erupting. Had I known what was in store that day, I wouldn't have brought her with me. When one lives with an abusive, alcoholic, narcissist one has to learn to deal with a Dr. Jekyll/Mr. Hyde personality.

Although I knew this concept deep down inside, I was not mature enough to understand the ramifications. So, as a person who tries to see the good in people, I took a chance and brought Lynda for a visit. Jim must have been watching for us to come inside. I had just taken my shoes off while Lynda was in the porch with hers on. He came running through the door wielding a hammer like a madman. My heart jumped up in my throat as I saw him coming at me, screaming something about what I had said about Ruby's hair in rollers. Lynda and I ran out of the house—her with shoes on and I in bare feet—over the gravel road, to her house about five minutes away.

My heart was racing and my body was stricken with fear. Lynda's family were horrified when they learned what had happened. They wanted to keep me and I desperately wanted to stay with them in a home where it was welcoming and loving. Jim, however, had contacted the RCMP. They contacted Lynda's father and informed him that if he did not send me back home he would be charged. Word of this incident spread rapidly around Burnside and the surrounding little communities. As the saying goes, the cat was out of the bag.

I walked into the kitchen and was mortified to see the RCMP officer and Jim sitting at the table reading pages from my diary. I was a promiscuous teenager so one can only imagine the horror I felt as I saw them discover my deepest personal secrets.

Although I don't remember the issue at hand on that particular evening when Jim was in another drunken rage, I do recall the terror I felt. I searched the phone book, desperate to find someone to help me get out of that house. I couldn't find anything to help. The "system" had failed me. Follow up with social workers in Newfoundland should have been arranged by the Ontario CAS when I was placed back with Jim and returned to Newfoundland. As a child I was, once again, left to suffer more trauma, without any escape.

I was trapped. There was nowhere for me to go. I decided I would make the best of it, counting down the days until I could get away from Jim's control. I tried so very hard to be a good kid. If I was good—even perfect—Jim would have no reason to pick on me. I excelled in school and became a people pleaser. However, no matter how hard I tried there was no pleasing him. He managed to pick apart even my best efforts. I craved his approval.

He rarely gave it. It was a challenge to get on his good side. Try as I might, I never knew what to expect from him. I learned to read him, a skill that would serve me well as I pursued a career as a counsellor later in life.

In September 1972 I went to Grade 9 at Holy Cross Central High in Eastport. It took me away from the turmoil at home; school always was an escape for me. I made good friends in high school and participated in extracurricular activities like Speech Club, Drama Club, Student Council and Yearbook Committee, to name a few. I worked hard, studied a lot and got really good grades.

Attending school in Eastport was a good experience. I was popular and was even crowned Miss Central High one year and Carnival Queen the next. I fit in well with the other students without having to compromise my values, unlike my experience in London. The kids in Eastport were behind the times—in a good way—when it came to experimenting with illegal drugs. I was happy to be in a healthy environment, as least in school, if not at home.

I was the new kid in town, which sparked interest from some of the guys; I dated a few. One in particular, Frank, was crazy about me. He had bought me a ring but I didn't give him the opportunity to give it to me. His aftershave was a turnoff, so I broke up with him.

Bill, whom I first laid eyes on in August of 1972, was still in the back of my mind, and I couldn't let him go. I fell in love with him the moment I saw him. I was with Lynda at Benger's Hangout in Eastport. She had briefly dated Bill but was no longer interested in him. We sat on a bench beside a large window at the front of the Hangout. Bill stepped out of a car wearing a red plaid lumber jacket, and blue jeans which were partially tucked inside his tan work boots.

"Hide me," Lynda said as she slid behind me on the bench.

I reached in front of her and peered out the window. I couldn't take my eyes off him. He slowly walked across the parking lot, his long blonde curls blowing in the soft breeze. This moment in time is forever etched in my mind. He walked into the Hangout and bought a pack of cigarettes and, just as quickly, disappeared back into the car. Every part of my body tingled. I knew he was the one, and I was determined to have him.

My friends and I dropped numerous hints to Bill when we started school in September. He was shy and had very little confidence. I was quite the opposite, and I began to wonder if he'd ever show an interest in me.

Finally, one day a bunch of us were hanging out in front of the Eastport Post Office when Bill made his move. He took my mitten. When we stopped running after each other and he gave the mitten back to me, we started walking to a teen dance at the Royal Canadian Legion. It was December 1, 1972. He was sixteen and I was fourteen. I will always remember when he reached out and caught hold of my hand. It felt magical. There was a huge puddle of water in the middle of the road, so Bill walked on one side and I on the other, and when we arrived at the Legion we weren't holding hands. Hence, we each paid our own way into the dance. I still tease Bill about letting go of my hand because he didn't want to pay for me, as was the tradition at the time.

Our first date was everything I expected it to be, with one exception. I had just broken up with Frank. He was not over me and, of course, blamed it on Bill. He told everyone he was going to beat Bill up after the dance. This put a little damper on our evening, but we danced and enjoyed every minute. I had to head home after the dance as there was a ride waiting for the people from Burnside. Bill decided to stay behind and face Frank, and I was concerned about him. When I arrived home, he phoned to let me know nothing happened. Frank changed his mind.

Although Jim wouldn't allow me to date and I knew he'd be angry if he found out, I continued to secretly see Bill. Jim's sister, my Aunt Lily, was often successful in getting on Jim's good side. She was my idol, a woman who was ahead of her time, very classy, strong, determined and assertive. I admired her and her attitude. She lived in Ontario and occasionally came to visit with my grandmother.

She visited at Christmas of 1972, and I encouraged her to ask Jim if he would permit me to have Bill come to visit. I thought that Aunt Lily could reason with him, as few could. Sure enough, to my delight, he agreed that Bill could visit.

As with most crushes and teenagers, it wasn't long before I was interested in dating other guys and there were other guys who were interested in me. But now I had a dilemma: if I broke up with Bill, Jim would be furious. He and Bill had connected, as they both liked to drink, so they would drink together in Jim's workshop. For this reason, I stuck with Bill and our love deepened.

Bill turned seventeen in January 1973 and got his driver's license shortly thereafter. This made seeing him so much easier, as his father would allow him to use his truck when he didn't need it. The eight-kilometre distance between where he lived in Eastport and my place in Burnside wasn't as big a barrier to seeing each other on the weekends.

Bill and I spent our breaks and lunches together when we were in school. In the evenings when I finished studying I'd phone Bill. Today we laugh about being on the phone for long periods and having to contend with interruptions from our neighbours. We had party lines in Eastport and Burnside, so when we heard a click we knew someone wanted to use the phone and we had to hang up.

Bill decided he wanted me to meet his family, and I was keen to meet them too. His family had heard the rumour about Jim chasing me with the hammer. I guess you could say that I had gotten a bad reputation, as gossip had spread about the incident. This was unknown to me and, to my delight, I believe I proved some people wrong. Apparently, there was a discussion about me between Bill and his family. Bill's father, a quiet and reserved man, overheard some of this discussion. He walked into the room and asked what was going on. After Bill explained that I wasn't who some were saying I was, his father told them all to stop the discussion, to invite me to supper and then they could all judge for themselves. I had no knowledge of this exchange at the time. I'm glad I didn't as I would have been very nervous to meet the family.

As was customary in outport Newfoundland, Bill's mother made salads for Sunday supper. His father, being traditional, preferred salt fish. I was served salads and cold beef, which I really enjoyed. Mr. Samson, whom I was sitting beside, asked if I would like some salt fish. I love salt fish and would never pass up the opportunity to enjoy some. Apparently, after I had eaten and left their home, Mr. Samson voiced his approval of me. This was the beginning of a wonderful relationship with Bill's family.

Because Bill lived within walking distance of our high school, he went home for lunch. Students from Burnside were bussed to school and had to bring a lunch. I, however, was quickly spoiled by Bill's mother. I ate lunch there every school day. I'm not a fan of leftovers, especially with gravy, so when Mrs. Samson was serving leftovers, she would make a special lunch for me—often a hamburger and French fries. She always made me feel special.

Things were still tense at my house. Jim's behaviour hadn't changed, and the drinking continued. He still wanted control. School nights were meant for studying, and I didn't waver from my studies. It was important for me to be as perfect as I could possibly be. If I was a "good" girl I may avoid Jim's anger, especially when he had been drinking.

As I reflect on my life, trying to determine when my body started to show effects of the constant stress I was under, my mind goes to an incident on the school bus in Grade 10 when I became short of breath and felt faint. I didn't understand what was happening, so I went to the doctor and was advised to carry a paper bag with me at all times. When this feeling overtook me I was to breathe into the paper bag in order to slow down my breathing. Bill became my rescuer and carried the paper bag with him at all times. I now realize I was actually experiencing anxiety which, in turn, caused me to hyperventilate.

I really looked forward to going to teen dances on the weekends. Ruby was not allowed to give me permission to go out; I had to ask Jim's permission to go to a dance. Each time I had to ask him I felt that he got great pleasure in being the "controller." I wanted to rebel, as that part of me wasn't "straightened out" as he had so smugly told me. The difference was that I could now keep the rebel in me under control. I saw an end in sight. I had school to keep me busy, and I had Bill.

Bill was always on mind. How many times did I write "Debbie loves Bill" on my schoolbooks! I have fond memories of Bill visiting me in Burnside. We would get cozy on the daybed in the kitchen. Jim and Ruby would be watching TV in the living room which, thankfully, was separated from the other living areas. Bill and I would hang out with Nannie in the kitchen, which was always a pleasant place to be. Nannie created an atmosphere of safety, but I could never let my guard down as I knew Jim was in the next room and all hell could break loose at any time.

Eventually, Nannie met Bill's family. She felt comfortable with Mrs. Samson and would often accompany Bill and I for a visit with her. It was comforting and validating to hear my grandmother tell Mrs. Samson about the abusive environment we lived in. She was talking about her own son, so, as I listened to her with admiration, I knew I wasn't imagining things. I knew Jim's behaviour was real and that someone else understood. I also learned it was okay to speak up and tell the truth. This woman taught me so much, and I will be forever grateful for a grandmother who was advanced in her thinking. She didn't sugar-coat it; she said it like it was.

When I visited Bill's home I felt safe and comfortable. This was a place where I could let my guard down and relax. I could be me. Mrs. Samson was a funny lady and always made me laugh. She spent a lot of time cooking. I can picture her, apron on, coming out of the "slut's hole" (as she called it)—her disorganized pantry. One never knew what was going to come out of her mouth, and Bill inherited her sense of humour. It was heartwarming and quite the opposite of the atmosphere at my house. I dreaded going back to Burnside.

Bill was a year behind me in school. In the 1970s there was no extra help for someone who had difficulty learning. Bill is an extremely smart guy, but school just wasn't for him. He struggled through the best he could. His parents were concerned about what he would do in his future without an education. Bill's sister, Barb, came home for a visit from Labrador City in March 1974. Bill's family convinced him to quit school and go to Labrador with her because it was easy to pick up a job there. Within a few months he found employment with the Iron Ore Company of Canada.

I was heartbroken when he went away, but I looked forward to his Sunday night phone calls and weekly letters. To deal with missing Bill I immersed myself in my studies and engaged in activities which kept my mind occupied. I counted down the days until I would see Bill again. I kept a very busy schedule, never having time for loneliness or boredom.

Home Economics was a class which really interested me, especially when we were taught to sew. I enjoyed making my own clothes. Ruby and Nannie were quite talented in this area, so what I didn't learn in school they taught me at home. Nannie showed me her quilt-making skills. Because she was nearly blind and could no longer sew, it brought her great joy that I took an interest in making quilts. Ruby was an incredibly talented crocheter and knitter. She patiently taught me to do both. During my remaining time in high school, with Bill away in Labrador, I created many items in my spare time. I'm grateful that I learned these skills, as they've served me well throughout my life.

I counted down the days until I would see Bill when he came home for a visit in June. Although he was only away for three months, it seemed like forever. To my surprise he brought an engagement ring with him. I was only sixteen but, yes, we got engaged! My friends at school told me it wouldn't last, but here we are forty-six years since that June day, and he is still by my side.

My studying efforts paid off, and I passed Grade 10 with straight As. I worked extremely hard to get these good grades although, at times, it was difficult. Others in my class criticized me for my determination to succeed, and it was a challenge to avoid the crowd, but I had made success my goal and was determined not to let anyone or anything get in the way.

To my delight, Bill bought me a plane ticket to visit him in Labrador City during the summer of 1974. I met some of his friends and saw where he worked. The trip made me more excited than ever, as I planned to move to Labrador City with Bill as soon as I finished high school the following year. Not only was I counting down the days until I could be with Bill, I was also counting down the days until I would get away from my so-called "home."

I thought my final year of high school would never end. Sunday night chats with Bill helped me see a light at the end of the tunnel. June and graduation rolled around, and Bill surprised me a couple days prior to graduation when he showed up, unannounced. To my disappointment, Jim would not attend my extra-curricular events. Nannie, Ruby and Bill came to my high school graduation, but Jim would not go. I was the class valedictorian, and I will never understand how a parent could not want to be there for such a momentous occasion. The only event he ever showed up for was a Lion's Club Speak Off that I participated in. I so desperately wanted him to take pride in my efforts, but he just wasn't interested.

Bill had purchased my plane ticket to Labrador City months prior to graduation. I finished public exams on July 4 and was on the plane to Labrador on the sixth. I could hardly contain myself; finally, the day I had dreamed of was here. Joy, a friend who graduated with me, accompanied me on the flight. Her boyfriend was also working at the Iron Ore Company in Labrador City. Joy and I had counted down the last few days together.

The "diary" incident had played on my mind the remaining time I lived under Jim's roof. He had searched my bedroom and found it when I ran out of the house in the hammer incident. It felt as though he was holding it over my head, and I was determined to take it out of his control. I searched his bedroom and found my diary. Before I left the house for the airport to catch my flight to Labrador, I spoke to Nannie about my concerns. As always, she was on my side. I told her I was going to burn it, and she felt it was the right thing to do. I appreciated her support. With trembling hands and a pounding heart, I brought the diary down to the kitchen, opened the cover of the woodstove and watched it burn. I was terrified Jim would catch me, as he was in the next room. If he knew, he didn't say a word. The incident was never again mentioned to me.

I was on my own at the tender age of sixteen. I was finally free to make my own decisions and free of Jim's control. He tried to run my life, but I wouldn't let him. I desperately wanted to be on my own and prove I was my own person who was able to fight for my dreams and make them come true.

To have peace, I had no choice but to refrain from arguing with him, but there was still a fighter in me. His behaviour was irrational and I knew it. Out of a horrific home life I learned to think for myself; I was resilient, yet I was angry. That anger fuelled me and enabled me to stand up for myself; it gave me determination. Once I began to learn about childhood abuse, neglect and trauma, I understood what the problem was. It was not my fault, and I was not crazy.

I was in such a rush to get out of Jim's house that I didn't consider my future career. My only goal was to go to Labrador with Bill. So, here I was fresh out of high school and looking for a job. Within a few days I began as a cashier at The Gift Box, a local jewelry and gift store.

Bill and I lived with his sister, Barb, for a few months until we had enough money to move into an apartment together. As I really missed Nannie, we decided she would visit. Just before we moved to our apartment, her and Bill's mother flew to Labrador, and it was great to have their company. A few days after Nannie's arrival I noticed she was different; her speech was slurred and her face drooped on one side. Further tests revealed she had suffered a stroke. She shortened her visit, as it was in her best interest to return to Newfoundland. She was assessed at the hospital in Gander and, thankfully, there were no after-effects. I was sad to see Nannie go back to Newfoundland, but I knew it was the right thing to do. This episode was an eye-opener for me. I was saddened as I realized that Nannie's age wasn't in her favour. I worried that she would have another stroke which could cause a more serious outcome.

My job at The Gift Box was short lived. I was working with the manager and another cashier on a particularly busy evening. Three of us were using the cash register. When the cash was counted at the end of the evening, we were short approximately $20. The manager told us we would each have to put our share in to make up the loss and, me being me, I told her we would have to divide it three ways, as all of us were using the cash. She told me she didn't make mistakes so it would just be divided two ways. I argued with her. She told me that I better be quiet or else! I said that if "or else" meant I was fired, then I quit.

With that, I walked out.

I received a call from the owner of the business the following morning. She apologized and offered me my job back, but I politely told her I was not interested in working with their unreasonable manager. I was proud that I stood up for myself.

Within a couple of weeks, I found another job at a drugstore. It helped pay the bills, but I knew I couldn't continue working in retail. Living in an isolated mining town made it a challenge to further my education, but I was determined to find a way to develop my skills. Office administration was of interest to me so I enrolled in a typing course and an accounting course in night school. The following year, I was offered the opportunity to teach the typing course to adults, which I enjoyed. I maintained my job at the drugstore where I had been promoted to head cashier.

It Was No Honeymoon

Jim said I wasn't permitted to get married until I turned eighteen. Bill and I would have gotten married on my eighteenth birthday, August 25, 1976, but it was a Thursday so we chose the twenty-seventh, a Saturday. My gut was telling me not to marry him, but I didn't listen. Truthfully, I didn't know how to stop the wedding. The invitations were in the mail, I had made my wedding dress, the venue was booked, the band was hired, the flowers were ordered. Deep down in my heart I knew I wasn't happy, but I hoped it would change.

As the saying goes, out of the frying pan into the fire. As is often the case, I left one alcoholic home for another. When I settled into life in Labrador City, I was surprised to discover how much and how often Bill drank. I spent many nights alone while he was at the club. I would call and ask him to come home, but he usually didn't show up when he said he would. When he did come home he was often so drunk that he just fell asleep. Bill was a different type of drunk than Jim. While Jim was violent and abusive, Bill was fairly quiet and tired.

I had some insight into Bill's drinking when he was in Labrador and I was finishing high school in Eastport. Time and again I called his sister's looking to speak to him, but he wasn't home. I would leave a message for him to call me back, but the call often didn't come until the next day. I would later learn he had been out drinking. I repeatedly asked him to stop drinking or slow it down, but he was in denial. He would promise to stop but inevitably fall off the wagon.

I had no idea what alcoholism was, and I grew more and more frustrated with Bill's drinking. I was tired of his empty promises, so I threatened, begged, yelled, fought and nagged him to stop. I was desperate. When Bill was intoxicated, I often took my frustrations out on him. He attempted to rationalize his drinking, and "Everyone else does it" was at the top of the list. He was right, as he surrounded himself with others who drank as much, or more, than him. He tried to convince me that he could stop whenever he wanted but he just didn't want to. He compared himself to his friends—"I'm not as bad as this person or that person." He rationalized his drinking by citing the fact that he still had a job. Even a snowmobile DUI was justifiable in Bill's mind.

I was in love with Bill, and I didn't want to give up on our marriage but as his drinking escalated, I had doubts. I signed us up for a Marriage Encounter Weekend, sponsored by the Catholic Church. We were encouraged to talk to each other and were assigned activities which helped us communicate. I poured out my concerns in our writing assignments, and Bill seemed to understand. We stayed at a hotel where everything was provided for us so there would be no outside interference. As fate would have it, one of Bill's drinking buddies— whose wife had also signed them up in an effort to save their marriage—was also there. They got together and drank despite the fact it was supposed to be an alcohol-free weekend.

Attending night school while working full time presented its own challenges but it paid off. I landed my first clerical job with Underwriter's Adjustment Bureau. During my interview I was asked if I intended to become pregnant within a year (that type of questioning would be illegal today). I wanted a new career so badly, so I told them I didn't plan to have children within the foreseeable future. With this in the back of my mind, I waited to get pregnant.

I began grasping at straws and was determined to "fix" Bill. After five years of marriage, I became pregnant. I had not wanted to have children but eventually changed my mind. Subconsciously I hoped that having a child would make Bill see the light. What it did, however, was put additional responsibilities on my shoulders. As Bill's tolerance for alcohol increased he became less and less dependable.

Sometime during my pregnancy, David came to Labrador City to look for work; he stayed at our house. Eventually, his pregnant girlfriend also came to stay with us. Being pregnant, having all the responsibility of a household and working full time was sometimes a lot to bear. David, however, did not make the situation any easier.

Something aroused me from my sleep one evening. As I crept downstairs I saw David's girlfriend sobbing at the table. After calming her down, she was able to tell me that David was in our rec room with another woman. I was furious! How dare he bring his pregnant girlfriend to my home and then have the nerve to cheat on her right under her nose! And in my home! I marched downstairs, flung open the rec room door and shouted, "Get that slut out of my house immediately!" It wasn't long before a taxi pulled up and she left. To this day, I have no idea who the woman was.

David and his girlfriend broke up, and she went home to have her baby. I remained friends with her and visited with her and my niece until she started seeing another man. It was then that she refused to allow her daughter to have any contact with David's side of the family.

Before David moved into an apartment with a friend, he was looking around my house for a cassette tape. He couldn't find a blank one so he took the only cassette of our wedding and taped over it. It felt like a slap in the face, and it was many years before I got him to admit that he did it. I let him stay at my home and he treated me with absolutely no respect. I should have realized that I was dealing with another "Jim," but it would take many more years to see the light.

Bill injured his ankle at work, which required him to be off work for rest and, eventually, surgery for torn ligaments. With more time on his hands, Bill's drinking escalated.

Bill was at the hospital for Lisa's birth. It was a long, hard labour which began on Friday, March 13. I didn't want my baby to be born on Friday the thirteenth, although I'm not a superstitious person. I recall being in extreme pain, but as the large, black clock on the wall hit one minute past midnight, I said to Bill, "Yay, our baby won't be born on the thirteenth!" Bill was with me every step of the way. I held his arm tightly and screamed through the pain. This was the supportive man I ached for.

On Saturday, March 14, 1981, at 1:39 a.m. our beautiful blue-eyed baby girl was born. She was perfect. I counted her fingers and toes, and I smile to myself as I remember there were ten of each. Her tiny, precious face looked even smaller under her massive head of black hair. Bill wanted to name her Lisa Dawn. I wanted to name her Melissa Jodie. We compromised, somewhat, and nicknamed her Lisa, which is short for Melissa.

I had a retained placenta, so Dr. McCarthy manually removed it. He told us that he hoped he'd gotten all of it, but he couldn't be certain because he had pieced it together in a tray. Within a few hours after Lisa's birth I began hemorrhaging. I had no idea what was happening and nervously pushed the buzzer for the nurse. I began to panic as I felt the blood flow from me like a raging river. I was rushed to the OR for an emergency D&C.

I spent a couple of weeks in the hospital and, despite this being my first baby, I knew something didn't feel quite right. I had started breastfeeding and was doing well with it. A few days after being discharged from hospital, I was passing large blood clots and became sicker. Upon visiting my doctor, he discovered I had an infection which required me to be readmitted to hospital for another D&C.

I was the only patient they would admit to the hospital so, despite the fact that I was breastfeeding, I could not bring Lisa with me. As I speak of this now it seems surreal; not allowing a nursing mother and her newborn back in the hospital together! Bill was incapable of caring for Lisa on his own, and we had no family to depend on. Thankfully, my friend, Cynt, came to the rescue. Bill made daily trips to the hospital to retrieve my breast milk.

I was exhausted when I left the hospital. Lisa had developed colic and cried constantly. I sat on the bed with her in my arms at a total loss and almost at the end of my rope. I had asked Ruby to come to Labrador City to help out, but she wouldn't. Although it was against my better judgement, Bill and I decided to return to Newfoundland. Ruby took Lisa during the night while I caught up on some much-needed rest. I'm sure I would have been back in the hospital had we not made this move.

I slowly began to regain my strength, but I was far from back to normal when my three-month maternity leave was over. Three-month maternity leave—absurd! Because I was unwell, I had to give up breastfeeding. I was mentally and physically exhausted and had to take my three-month-old to a babysitter. I went back to work at Underwriter's Adjustment Bureau, but I was not happy. I needed to be with my baby girl.

The local newspaper ran an advertisement for a part-time lottery ticket sales distributor with the Atlantic Lottery Corporation (ALC). It sounded like it would satisfy my desire to spend more time with Lisa and be fulfilling for me to work outside the home. I applied and, as luck would have it, the job was mine.

The position with ALC was convenient because I could choose my work hours. I received lottery tickets from ALC and distributed them to retailers in Labrador City and Wabush biweekly. It meant handling large amounts of cash. In the evening after Lisa was in bed, I prepared the required reports for ALC. The following day I did the banking and returned unsold tickets. I enjoyed this position and held it for five years.

In 1983 I received a call from Avery Adjusting Ltd. offering me a temporary clerical position. They were willing to accommodate my job with ALC. After some hesitation, I accepted the offer. My experience with Underwriter's Adjustment Bureau made the transition to Avery Adjusting a natural fit. I liked working in the insurance claims field, and I even took a couple of Insurance Institute of Canada courses to enhance my skills.

Because of his drinking, Bill wasn't an involved parent when Lisa was little. But I loved being a mom. Playing with Lisa enabled me to enjoy the things I had missed out on without fear of violence. It was like having a second chance at childhood.

After Lisa was born I vowed I'd never have another child. My friends told me I'd soon forget what labour was like, but I have not forgotten to this day. Despite my assertion, within a couple years we decided to try getting pregnant again.

I was into my first trimester when we went camping with Bill's sister and some friends. My nephew and his little friend were playing with an axe even though they were told not to, as they were too young. While sitting in our camper, I heard a lot of screaming and commotion.

"Find the top of Cory's finger!" is etched in my mind.

He was rushed to the hospital for surgery.

The evening of Cory's accident I felt a hard pain in my lower back. Thinking it wasn't anything to be concerned about but erring on the side of caution, I went to the hospital. The doctor did a number of pregnancy tests—a negative one and then a positive one, then another negative, and so on. It was overwhelming. The doctor explained I had a missed abortion, a term that I had never heard. I was admitted for a D&C. Although there is no way of knowing, I've always felt that the fright I got when Cory's finger got chopped off with the axe was the cause of my miscarriage. Science may not agree with my theory.

I sensed that miscarriage was a taboo subject. Well-meaning people attempted to comfort me by saying, "It wasn't meant to be," "Everything happens for a reason," "At least you weren't too far along," or "At least you can get pregnant." I know they were trying to be helpful, but I received the message that I should just suck it up and move on. As I did with most ordeals, I stuffed it deep down where I couldn't feel it. It was many years later, in therapy, that I allowed myself to grieve the loss of my baby that could have been.

Nannie was my world, but I knew I had to prepare myself to lose her. We must face reality, especially when a loved one reaches their eighties. She had a couple more strokes, and it was obvious she was deteriorating. Although I started grieving in my own way prior to her death, there was no way to totally prepare myself for the call that she had passed away. Bill stayed with Lisa while I flew to Newfoundland alone on December 23. The plane was full of young, jovial men singing Christmas songs on their way home for the holidays while I quietly wept and tried to avoid them.

The woman who loved me unconditionally was gone. She taught me to be a good person. She was my protector who gave of herself, never expecting anything in return. She showed me joy and humour, and she instilled a sense of pride in me. Nannie brought me to a place of worship where I found God. She is the person who gave me a love that endures, a love that has carried me through the most difficult days of my life and a love that showed me how to love others. As I write this tribute of Nannie today, tears well up in my eyes. I will miss her forever, but she lives on in my heart.

I have beautiful memories of my grandmother. Whenever I see a rose or lilac tree, I cannot walk by without stopping to smell the flowers. As I breathe in the aroma I feel my grandmother's presence and remember that her love still flows through me. It leaves me feeling peaceful. This woman is a part of me; she lives on through the virtues she instilled in me.

Upon my return home I called a friend Bill and I had been close with from when we arrived in Labrador City. She was very offish, leaving me puzzled. Her and her husband had been in our bridal party and us in theirs. It felt like we were being pushed away. No more invitations to play cards. No visits or phone calls. The friendship ended without explanation. Turns out that while I was attending Nannie's funeral, Bill had been drinking while visiting his sister, Barb. Because Bill was drunk, she and a friend went to our house and took Lisa and enough clothes until I came home. Our friends heard of this incident, and I can only assume they didn't want to associate with us because of it. They were the only non-drinking friends Bill associated with, which made matters worse, as he gravitated to his drinking buddies.

I was desperate to make Bill stop drinking but it felt like I was losing the battle as his denial intensified. I talked to our family doctor who offered to make arrangements for Bill to go to rehab at the Donwood Institute in Toronto. I ran this idea by Bill, but he was unwilling at the time.

The straw that broke the camel's back was when I came home from work and found Bill passed out on the chesterfield; I couldn't wake him. Lisa, just two years old, was playing with her toys. I was sickened as I considered what could have happened to her. Finally, in a last-ditch effort to help him, I gave him an ultimatum: seek help or I would leave and take Lisa. I had made this threat before, but this time he took me seriously. In March 1984, Bill, although resistant, went to treatment for four weeks.

When Bill returned from Donwood he was a new man, and an enormous weight was lifted off my shoulders. He went to Alcoholics Anonymous (AA) meetings and suddenly realized he had no friends. The old drinking buddies were just that, drinking buddies. They no longer visited because there was no booze. Bill began making new friendships within the AA community.

I had started a new clerical job with the United Steelworkers International Office. It was four hours a day, Monday to Friday. An even better aspect of the job was that I had every summer off. This was the job I had been searching for. It fulfilled my desire to spend more time with Lisa and my need to have something for me. It also enabled me to continue my part-time position with the Atlantic Lottery Corporation.

I met Salome, the secretary with the United Steelworkers Local 5795, at the Union Office, and she introduced me to Al-Anon, a program of recovery for people who are affected by another person's drinking. Salome became a true friend. She's one of those rare people you find an instant connection with and is always there for you through the good and the bad. She became one of the family, and I knew she would never let me down. C.S. Lewis says it well: "Friendship is born at that moment when one person says to another, 'What! You too? I thought I was the only one.'" Our friendship has survived the test of time. Salome is there for me today, as she was when I first met her.

Bill and I decided it was the right time to have another baby, which meant I had to overlook my last two pregnancies. If I didn't, I would have never gotten pregnant for the third time. We excitedly awaited our new arrival in April 1985.

In the '80s, the practice at Donwood was to give patients Antabuse, a drug which causes a bad reaction if you drink alcohol. I was delighted that Bill was taking this drug because I had not yet gained trust in him. Having him take Antabuse each day was like having added insurance. To be certain he took the pill, each night I got it ready for him. One night, I had placed Bill's Antabuse and my prenatal vitamin on the table. I then went to the bottom of the steps and called Bill to come downstairs to take his pill. Without paying attention to what I was doing, I went back to the table and took what I though was the vitamin. It was too late; the pill was gone. I had taken Antabuse!

As the pill slipped down my throat I realized what I had done. I panicked! My thoughts ran wild. What about my unborn baby? I was so scared. With trembling hands, I dialled the hospital. The doctor on call assured me there was no need to be concerned. I was so relieved that I just sat and cried. I've often told this story as an illustration of my codependency. In Melody Beattle's book *Codependent No More: How to Stop Controlling Others and Start Caring for Yourself*, she writes, "We rescue people from their responsibilities. We take care of people's responsibilities for them." It has taken me much hard work to unlearn these behaviours.

As was the case with my first pregnancy, I went past my due date. I decided to work until the baby was born and recall excitedly leaving work on a Monday afternoon knowing that we would have a new baby the following day. In the back of my mind I thought of my previous pregnancies but made every effort to push away the anxiety.

April 23, 1985, without any complications and an easy labour, our beautiful baby boy was born. Bill and I were ecstatic. Our little family was now complete.

Bill's family originates from Flat Island, a resettled community in Bonavista Bay. When the island was a bustling fishing settlement, the name Bill Samson was commonplace; so much so that in order to distinguish them, they were given nicknames. I have a fond memory of Bill's mother rhyming the list of Bills: Gunner Bill, Midder Bill, Billy Field, Bill Lower Island, Brother Bill and Bill Shoal Tickle.

While walking across the garden at Bill's parents' just after I started dating him, I met a much older Bill Samson. He had owned a general store on Flat Island and was visiting Bill's parents from Mount Pearl. I've always remembered his request: "If you ever have a little boy, will you promise me that you'll name him Bill Samson to carry on the tradition?" At that time there were only two Bill Samsons remaining, as the others had all passed away. When our son was born, there was only one Bill Samson remaining, and it was important to us to keep the tradition alive; therefore we named our little boy William. Our plan was not to shorten his name to Bill as it would be too confusing to have two Bill Samsons in our immediate family.

Bill had remained sober since his return from treatment at Donwood, just over a year prior to William's birth. Against my advice, he had stopped taking Antabuse. After Bill left William and I at the hospital, he picked up a case of beer. Trying to prove that he could be a social drinker, he drank part of a bottle when he arrived home. I was disappointed when Bill told me he had drank, but he assured me he could control it. I wanted to believe him, but I had a better understanding of addiction, and I wasn't convinced. Al-Anon taught me to let go of my obsession with Bill's alcoholism so, for my own sanity, I had to leave it to Bill to figure out if he could be a social drinker. Al-Anon taught me to detach, with love, from Bill's alcoholism. I had to allow him to learn from his mistakes and concentrate on my own behaviour to try to make myself a better person.

As was the case when both of my children were born, I was entitled to three months maternity leave. Because I had summers off at my job, I returned to work in September, which gave me a few more weeks with my boy. It was not nearly enough though. William was a colicky baby. Our precious little boy wailed in pain for hours at a time. I felt powerless. Neither home remedies nor prescriptions alleviated his extreme discomfort. As he screamed, I walked the floors and cried the tears that he didn't. It was a gut-wrenching experience. Neither William nor I got proper sleep.

Lisa is four years older than William, and she has memories of his non-stop crying episodes. She tells the story of coming downstairs to the living room and seeing me crying while William was crying in his brown cradle beside me. She remembers wanting to tip the cradle over, as a four-year-old would, to stop his crying. She also remembers the one and only night we spent in our new camper before we sold it because William cried the entire night (as he did most nights).

Our darling little boy had colic until he was almost two years old, so our family doctor made an appointment with a pediatrician at the Janeway Children's Hospital in St. John's. While we sat on a waiting list, our precious boy continued to suffer. The feeling of powerlessness over this dreadful condition is something I will never forget. Miraculously, within days of receiving an appointment with the pediatrician, William's pain ended. It was overnight—instant. His pain left and his suffering was over. Our whole family felt a load lifted off our shoulders.

Bill's alcohol relapse began the night of our son's birth and spiralled out of control again. One night we went to our neighbour's anniversary party. I came home alone early because Bill wasn't ready to leave the party. Late into the night I heard a loud bang outside the door. When I went to investigate, I found Bill passed out on the steps. He was so intoxicated that he had trouble walking, his speech was slurred and he was incoherent. With great difficulty, I got him into the house and onto the chesterfield where he slept off his drunken stupor.

Part of me was sad and another part of me was angry. I realized there was a high probability that a recovering alcoholic would relapse because I had learned that alcoholism is an illness. With a much better grasp of addiction, I could offer more compassion to Bill, so we had a frank conversation regarding his relapse the following morning. He also began feeling the effects of alcohol withdrawal. Reluctantly, he acknowledged he would have to be hospitalized in order to begin a new road to recovery. He was admitted to the Captain William Jackman Memorial Hospital for a few days to help with detox. He was given passes to attend AA meetings in the evenings, which gave him an opportunity to reconnect with AA members he had lost touch with during his relapse.

Those early days of sobriety were challenging for Bill, and he needed support. Both of us are grateful to our long-time friend, Alvin, who took

Bill under his wing during this vulnerable period. Alvin owned a cabin at Albert Lake, a short distance from Labrador City, where he and Bill spent a lot of time. Eventually, Bill decided to build a cabin for us next door to Alvin's. This project was a great distraction for Bill. All of their spare time was devoted to construction at the cabin, which kept Bill away from the bottle.

The cabin project was put on hold when winter set in and was completed the next fall. By this time Bill was building a good foundation for his new way of life. He surrounded himself with new—sober—people who were in recovery.

Immersed in Recovery

Bill and I immersed ourselves in the Twelve Step community. Bill attended AA meetings regularly, while I went to Al-Anon. Sunday night AA meetings were "open" meaning anyone from the general public could attend. The open meeting provided an opportunity for Bill and me to learn and grow together.

As is the practice in AA, Bill became a sponsor of others who were new to the program. These individuals often came to our home and, on occasion, both Bill and I were able to help others through our own experiences. To know that we made a difference in someone else's life is heartwarming and rewarding. Over the years Bill and I have heard from numerous people we helped along the way. One such person sent this very thoughtful message to us:

Hey Debbie. I am passing this message on to you for Bill. Well, can you imagine 33 years ago Bill S. became the messenger and Angel I so desperately needed when I was at the lowest point in my life? He was the first message of hope I was ever given that there was a way out for me. I still have the book he brought to me on his 12th *Step call. I have given much literature and books away since but I cannot part with that book,* Alone No More.

I believe he was a genius because the second call I made to AA he was ready and this time was just a short message that somebody will be by to pick me up around 7:30. My first meeting was January 3rd*, 1988 and life was never the same. Bill was the best sponsor I could ever have, to tell me the truth and not sugarcoat it; tough at times for sure, but gentle when I needed compassion. I remember our last chat before I moved to St John's. He told me I was going to be fine and I have always held on to his last words to me: if I ever started to believe I wasn't an alcoholic, to call him.*

You, too, Debbie, were the best co-sponsor a woman could have. I have always been grateful for Al-Anon sharing you with me because you had to cross a boundary to help me. You never ever made me feel less than, or ashamed of being an alcoholic. I knew I had a winner in you when you honestly said to me that you could have been me. That made it so much easier to trust you.

I'm the person I am today because of the solid bonds I was given in my early sobriety. I will never forget. I still believe in passing it on to the ones who are still suffering. I love you guys so much. I have had a lot of ups and downs but I know that if I was to die tomorrow I was given 33 years of blessings, brought by the means of you and Bill.

Take care and keep safe. I keep you in my heart and prayers always. Thank you for your love and support when I felt so unlovable. I love you guys.

I was gaining a better understanding of myself and how alcoholism had affected me. I attended Adult Children of Alcoholics (ACoA) and Co-Dependents Anonymous (CoDA) meetings, and I read countless self-help books. Charles Whitfield's *Healing the Child Within* was one of my first invitations to connect with and heal my wounded inner-child. It was profound to finally understand that the little girl inside me needed nurturing, and that I could connect with her and begin the healing process. I immersed myself in the workbook, eagerly doing all the recommended activities. It was a painful process. I had to grieve the loss of a childhood, of being forced to grow up too fast in order to survive. Among other things, I learned that I was a perfectionist, a people pleaser and a rescuer. It's been a lifetime of unlearning unhealthy behaviours.

As I continued to understand more about alcoholism and myself, I felt a desire to help others touched by this disease. I started an Alateen group for young people affected by others' drinking. Coming together with these teenagers to share their experiences and watch them gain strength and hope was a rewarding experience.

A large number of people in the communities of Labrador City and Wabush (Labrador West) suffered from alcohol and drug use/abuse, and there were few resources available locally for these individuals. A group of concerned citizens formed the Labrador West Alcohol & Drug Advisory Committee, which Bill and I became involved in. It was a way for us to give back to the community, and it provided a forum to bring positive change. We lobbied government for services and organized educational community events, and I eventually accepted the chairperson role of this committee. One of our proudest accomplishments was the establishment of a "Don't Drink & Drive Awareness Day Motorcade" which celebrated its thirtieth anniversary in 2019.

It was at an Al-Anon meeting in 1987 that I was introduced to Line (pronounced Lynn). I was baffled when she spoke because of her French accent and fast talking combined with Newfie slang. It often made me sit back and shake my head. It was months before I started to understand her. Being an identical twin whose sister died at birth left me with an emptiness I have trouble describing. It is a void that has been difficult to fill. Finding my "soul sister," Line, is the closest I'll ever come to having a sister. Line's unique dialect elicits laughter from those of us who know her well. While driving past a tabernacle in Corner Brook, she said, "Look at the ta-barn-a-cul." Her quirky sense of humour has brought much needed laughter to my life. It is said that laughter is the best medicine, and Line's ability to make me laugh has been one of the best "pills" I've had to swallow.

The Urban Dictionary describes an "unbiological sister" as: "Your best friend in the whole entire world!!!! You love each other like a sister. You guys have like the same exact personality and have so many inside jokes: You're just like twins. You think the same things, do the same things and love the same things! No one can replace them and everyone knows that you guys are best friends!" This defines my best friend, Line, better than any words I could use.

On November 17, 1987, the early days of our friendship, Line's husband Max died. Bill didn't know Line at the time and was out for a coffee after an AA meeting. When he called to let me know where he was, he mentioned that Max was killed in an accident. I couldn't believe what I was hearing. I asked Bill to come home with Lisa and William so I could go to be with Line. Our friendship strengthened through this tragedy. It was, obviously, an unimaginably difficult time for her as a widow with two small children. I spent time with her whenever I could.

When Max died, I had been struggling to quit my pack-a-day smoking addiction. It was socially acceptable to smoke in the 1980s, but Line didn't smoke. With so many smokers visiting Line, the cloud in the house was so heavy at times it was difficult to see across the room. Line's eyes became irritated, so we put up a "No Smoking" sign. If I could get through this tragedy without a cigarette then I could make it in any situation, and I have. I have remained a non-smoker to this day.

When Lisa and William were young we made annual trips to spend time with our families on the island portion of Newfoundland and Labrador. Visits to Burnside were generally tense, as Jim's alcoholism spiralled out of control. One such occasion was David's first wedding. Jim had been drinking, and no amount of pleading could convince him to attend the wedding. It put a damper on the whole event. I was unable to relax, especially in church because I was continually looking over my shoulder and expecting that Jim would stagger in at any moment. Jim's personality and addiction made his behaviour unpredictable, and he was difficult to read. We couldn't understand why he was acting as he did, and he offered no explanation.

The day following the wedding, Jim disclosed that he had been diagnosed with cirrhosis of the liver. His swollen abdomen was that of a severely malnourished man and the yellow discolouration in the whites of his eyes showed the severity of his disease. The doctor warned him that death was inevitable if he didn't stop drinking but the damage could be reversed if he quit. Throughout the next few years he struggled to maintain sobriety; he refused help and had many relapses.

I understand that Jim was, undoubtedly, struggling with his addiction, and coming to terms with a cirrhosis diagnosis was difficult for him. However, I can't help feeling annoyed that he, characteristically, ruined what should have been an enjoyable and memorable occasion.

David's wife, Barb, and I became close. Even though she has remarried, her and I are still the best of friends. She has a very special place in my heart, and we have a lot in common. When it comes my biological family and I'm questioning my memories, she provides me with much needed validation.

I created a Facebook page for my autobiography, and I occasionally post excerpts from my book in an effort to gauge how people felt about my writing. On one occasion I posted an excerpt which showed the reader my fear of Jim. Barb responded by saying that she knew that fear all too well. This validation meant a lot to me. As a victim of abuse, I've questioned myself and wondered if it was really that bad. I know in my heart that it was, but hearing it from someone who witnessed it first-hand helped to alleviate my doubts.

David and Barb had a beautiful daughter, Sarah, whom I treasured. Before they divorced we spent family vacations with them. Lisa is four years older than William, Sarah is four years younger than William. The three of them were like peas in a pod. We were all close at that time, like one would want a brother, sister and their family to be. After David and Barb divorced, he stayed in Newfoundland, and Barb took custody of Sarah and moved back to Labrador. We included Sarah in our family's life, such as weekend sleepovers with Lisa and William. As they grew into their teenage years and early twenties, Lisa and Sarah became like sisters, even looking very much alike. Unfortunately, Sarah has taken a self-destructive path we can't follow her on. I pray she will turn her life around. I've lost my special niece but I hang on to hope.

I am thankful our children have no memories of Bill drinking. It was a huge relief when Bill got sober, so much so that I learned to overlook his unchanged behaviours. Essentially, he had put the cork in the bottle but was experiencing a "dry drunk." I walked on eggshells so I wouldn't agitate him. He was irritable, easily annoyed, impatient and irresponsible, and he became defensive when I brought my concerns to his attention. In his mind he had quit drinking and he couldn't understand what else I expected from him.

I had made up my mind that I would no longer dance around the issue, so for the second time in our marriage I told him I couldn't stay if he didn't make changes. When he asked what he needed to change, I said I was tired of trying to "fix" him and that he'd have to figure it out himself. Bill wrote a list of things he thought he should change, and I would have written the exact list. The changes began immediately and he hasn't looked back. I now call him "the man of my dreams."

Bill and I became comfortable sharing our stories of how alcoholism touched our lives at AA, Al-Anon and Alateen meetings. We were often invited to talk at other places in the community. Although it was challenging to divulge our experiences, it was gratifying to know it could help others. A thank-you letter from the Labrador West Status of Women Council sums it up nicely: "Your open and intimate discussion of your life experiences created the atmosphere where the women felt comfortable discussing situations in their own families."

Fulfilling My Calling

I can't recall the first time I realized an inner calling to help others; it seemed to gradually sneak up on me. I do remember praying to find a way to fulfil this calling.

Accessing the education I required wasn't easy, as there was no university or college in Labrador City, and leaving home to attend school was out of the question because I had two small children. I trusted that something would come my way, and it did.

McMaster University offered a number of programs through distance learning, so I took a leap of faith and enrolled in the Addictions Studies Program. This was the beginning of many years of studying at the dining room table while the children were sleeping.

One day, I saw an ad for an Employee Assistance Program Coordinator in the paper. As fate would have it, I was about to select my next course from McMaster and had decided on Developing an Employee Assistance Program: Essential Aspects and Components. I applied for the position, went through the selection process and, to my overwhelming delight, was offered the position.

Although I was not familiar with Employee Assistance Programs (EAP) at the time, I immediately knew this was where I was meant to be. It's a program that offers confidential, short-term counselling, advisory and information services to employees and their family members to help them deal with personal difficulties such as addiction, grief and depression, just to name a few. The program also offers education and prevention programs in various areas of personal and lifestyle issues such as stress management, assertiveness training and parenting, etc.

On July 1, 1990, I began fulfilling my calling. When they asked how much I expected for a salary, I answered, "It doesn't matter; I just want to do this work and would do it for free if I have to." It was never about the money, it was about helping people.

It is challenging to maintain anonymity and confidentiality when you live in a small, isolated town where people know each other. When I was hired to develop the EAP, I knew employees would be skeptical about a program that was new and that I needed to develop trust in order for people to feel comfortable seeking help. I personally visited every work area and presented the EAP to employees. There were many questions and concerns, so I made every effort to alleviate those concerns.

Having lived and worked in Labrador City prior to being given the opportunity to develop this program, I had a pretty good understanding of what would and would not be acceptable to employees and their families. I realized the importance of having a place where people could go anonymously to seek the help they needed for personal problems. Hence, I set up my office away from the work site in an apartment building. There was no waiting room and no walk-ins. Clients were assured that no one other than me would ever know who came for assistance. With time, I established the necessary trust, and the program became extremely popular.

My job offered endless opportunities. I went to conferences all across Canada and training in the US. When I travelled, I took the whole family so we could make a vacation out of it. Bill, Lisa and William even went to McMaster University with me and stayed on campus. I'm forever grateful for a company that gave me the job of my dreams while supporting me to further my education.

My position allowed me to grow the EAP into a unique program that was featured in numerous places, included my employer's international magazine. My professor at McMaster, Dr. Rick Csiernik, included the program in a chapter of a book he wrote about EAPs in Canada.

As the needs of employees and their families became evident, I made every effort to accommodate them. We met this need by establishing a program (funded equally by the employees and employer) to help families experiencing hardship, often due to an ongoing medical issue. Wanting to make this program truly inclusive, I suggested we change the name to an

Employee and Family Assistance Program (EFAP). Family members had sought help from day one, but adding "Family" to the name showed that everyone was included.

Together with a committee of union and management representatives, we developed a Respectful Workplace Program. It became apparent that education and intervention was required because of harassment and disrespect in the workplace, so I took on the role of mediating such incidents.

With the ever-increasing demand for assistance, I needed to hire help, which is when Pam Meaney-Pieroway and Josephine Gaulton-Rowe came onboard. These ladies not only became my right hand, but also two of the most cherished friends one could hope to find. Our friendships flourish to this day.

I thrived as I was encouraged by my peers and superiors to take the program in any direction I felt beneficial to employees and their families. Since Labrador City is an isolated mining community, there were not as many services for individuals with personal problems as there are in larger centres. I offered various programs to anyone from the community including smoking cessation, stress management and parenting workshops, just to name a few. Teaming up with peers in the community to find creative solutions also produced many successful initiatives, such as a Debriefing Team to assist anyone in the community involved in a traumatic event.

Not long after being hired, I was informed by a local social worker that in order to practice counselling in Newfoundland and Labrador I was required to register with the Newfoundland & Labrador Association of Social Workers (NLASW). I was concerned about this as I am not a social worker. I was shocked when I called NLASW and explained my circumstances without using my name or my employer. The executive director of NLASW, without hesitation, called me by name and informed me who I was employed by. Apparently, I had been "reported" to the association for practicing counselling while not being registered with the NLASW. I felt betrayed by those very people I worked hand in hand with in our community. The more I thought about it, the more I realized they were just protecting their turf, so it was time I protected mine (although I never imagined I would have to do so).

I started by discussing my concerns with my boss. As always, he was extremely supportive. He wrote a letter to the NLASW stating that private employers had the right to hire whomever they wished and that the NLASW had no jurisdiction over my practice. It felt great to know that he had my back.

I was trained to be an Employee Assistance Professional, and my studies specifically educated me to do the job I was hired for. I was not a social worker, nor did I have a desire to be one, but the NLASW incident made me determined to prove myself. I went on to obtain designations as a Certified Employee Assistance Professional (CEAP) with the Employee Assistance Professionals Association, a Registered Professional Counsellor (RPC) and a Master Practitioner in Clinical Counselling (MPCC) with the Canadian Professional Counsellors Association. Even so, I would have to prove myself as a professional on many more occasions.

Tragedy Strikes

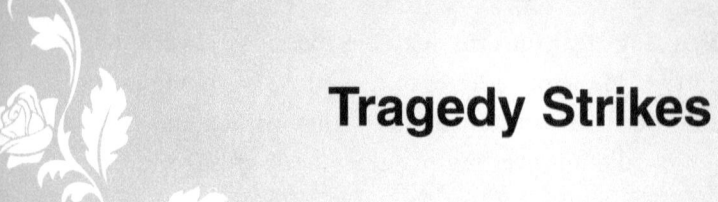

When we took Lisa and William to visit their grandparents in Newfoundland, the atmosphere at Bill's parents was relaxed and easy going. However, there was often tension at my parents' place. On one of our visits, Lisa and William were having fun and laughing heartily, as children do. Jim was watching TV and was annoyed that they were too loud.

"Can't you keep those kids quiet!" he yelled.

Then, to my shock, he slapped me across the back. I was furious, but I didn't want to rock the boat, so I bit my tongue. I was shaking from rage.

It took me years to realize that my family used me. When I gave money to them, it wasn't repaid. It bothered me, but I continued to allow them to walk over me.

In 1993, I attended a week-long inpatient treatment program for families of alcoholics at the Smith Clinic in Thunder Bay, Ontario. It was here that I learned, among other things, not to be a people pleaser. Phone calls were limited in the treatment centre so I hadn't spoken to my family in Newfoundland. On the flight back home, I used the Airfone to call Ruby and Jim.

"Dad's snowblower is broken. Can we borrow some money so he can get a new one?" was the first thing that came out of Ruby's mouth.

I was disgusted. With shaking hands and a pounding heart, I was able to say, "No, I'm sorry. I can't do that anymore." A part of me felt guilty, but the other part felt relieved that I wasn't allowing them to take advantage of me. Was it unreasonable to expect my parents to ask how I was doing when they hadn't heard from me for a while? I now understand that they weren't capable of such concern.

Jim was a know-it-all, a common characteristic of a narcissist. It gave me great satisfaction when I could prove him wrong. I knew my defiance made him furious. On one such occasion he told me that I shouldn't work because I was a tax burden to Bill. We argued this point, but as usual Jim wouldn't admit that he could be wrong. When tax time came I prepared the returns two ways, one where I filed as a single person and the other where Bill claimed me as a dependent. As I knew would be the case, it made financial sense for me to work. I smugly rubbed this in Jim's face.

Fur coats were fashionable in the 1990s, and I "thought" I wanted one. I later realized wearing the fur coat make me feel like a person who I am not. When I first got my coat I wore it to visit my parents and brother. The snide remarks about my coat were hurtful; they wouldn't let it go. I couldn't understand why they were so mean. It was a very long time before I realized that their hatefulness actually showed their envy. My realization was validated each time I achieved something, either tangible or intangible. Someone once said, "The jealous; when they can't cut it, they will try to cut you down." Since I'm now able to identify jealousy and envy, I try not to take it personally.

When our children got older we took memorable family vacations to different places. We occasionally went back to Newfoundland to visit family. One such trip was in the summer of 1995, and it was the last time I saw Jim alive. He had found sobriety and appeared to be very happy with Ruby. Jim was nice to me; the visit was pleasant. I left feeling there was hope for a healthy relationship with my parents.

Traumatic events have left permanent scars in my mind and on my brain, and I can vividly recall every minute of one such event. I was called out of a training session to take a phone call, so I instinctively knew something was wrong. I sat in shock as I listened to David say, "Dad and Mom were in an accident on the way to St. John's. Dad is dead. Mom is in ICU at the Health Science." My mind was racing. I couldn't concentrate. I collapsed in tears.

A couple of caring co-workers stepped in, comforted me and called Bill to take me home. When Lisa and William got home from school they knew something was wrong when they saw all the vehicles parked at our house. Our amazing friends were there to help us with all the arrangements, from making reservations to packing our suitcases. My friend, Salome, asked what we wanted to do about supper. I had taken out ground beef to make goulash, so she cooked it for us before we left on the evening flight to St. John's. It is the last time I ate goulash. I just can't bring myself to eat it; the memory is too overwhelming.

Upon arriving in St. John's, we rented a van and drove to the Health Science where we met David and his wife. CBC news was on in a waiting area, and my attention was immediately drawn to a report of the accident that showed the demolished cars. The other car had veered into Jim's lane, causing a head-on collision which left both men dead and their wives in hospital.

The image of Ruby in the ICU bed attached to tubes, drains and IV lines is gut-wrenching. She was most concerned that funeral arrangements needed to be made for Jim. She was not in good enough shape to attend the funeral, so she was denied closure. I felt helpless and heartbroken.

During the three-hour drive from St. John's we stopped by the RCMP headquarters in Clarenville to pick up Jim's personal belongings. My legs didn't want to move as I forced myself to walk around the building to look at the mangled wreck. No wonder he didn't survive—how could anyone have survived this horrendous collision?

As soon as Jim died, David began acting strangely. He was concerned that Jim's wallet wasn't with his personal belongings; apparently a neighbour had been at the accident scene and took the wallet for safe keeping. When we arrived in Burnside in the late evening hours, David insisted on waking the neighbours to get the wallet. I thought this to be odd but just overlooked it. Jim owned and operated a small engine repair business located next to their home. The moment we arrived at the house, David made a point of going to the repair shop. Again, it seemed odd but I overlooked it. In the following days, friends and neighbours came with sympathy cards. David took charge and opened the cards, which was also strange but I didn't think much of it either.

The final straw came when I went upstairs and discovered David going through the closet and bureaus in Jim and Ruby's bedroom. I insisted he stop looking through their personal belongings. He was frustrated that I intervened and, in no uncertain terms, told me to mind my own business. I felt strongly that David was denying Ruby the opportunity to deal with Jim's death in her own way when she was well again. I refused to back down from David, and our tempers flared. To my astonishment, he slapped me across the face. This infuriated me more, and I began swinging at him. We exchanged hurtful words, and he called out to Bill to get me out of there.

Bill, Lisa, William and I stayed at Bill's parents in Eastport until after the funeral because I did not feel welcome in Jim and Ruby's house. David had made it clear that he was taking control of the situation until Ruby was out of the hospital. He became someone who I didn't know; he became Jim. I was disappointed and hurt by his attitude. In my mind, because there were just the two of us, it made sense that we would both handle Ruby's affairs until she was able to do so herself. David was having no part of this and, because I had to return to Labrador, I left it in his hands. I did so, however, with a great deal of resentment.

Being the target of David's bullying after Jim's death left a sour taste in my mouth; I felt betrayed. Until then I'd had a fairly good relationship with him. We often talked about our childhoods, and we agreed that our home was abusive and dysfunctional. While his upbringing was not a bed of roses, I seemed to be Jim's most common target because I was the black sheep and rebel, whereas he was the favourite child.

When Jim died, David took possession of many of his belongings, one item being a pair of shoes. He literally stepped into Jim's leather shoes, and I instantly saw Jim's behaviour in my brother. Jim had tried to take away David's power on many occasions, and I can only assume that David saw his death as an opportunity to regain it. In doing so, he changed. Not only did I see him transform into a person exhibiting Jim's characteristics, but he suddenly defended Jim at every opportunity.

Ruby did the same. How could they suddenly put this man on a pedestal because he was dead? There was no way I was going to portray him as a saint just because he was dead, so David, Ruby and I clashed. I let my anger out at them and wrote letters telling them exactly how I felt. I had altercations with them. While visiting Ruby after the accident, she offered me the mustache cup. This was a unique antique china cup and saucer which was handed down through Nannie's family. As a child I was intrigued and amazed by the little semicircular ledge inside the cup. I would secretly take it off its home on the mantle in the living room, looking at the moon-shaped opening which served to keep moustaches dry while a man was drinking. I had never seen the cup in use so I would imagine a man drinking from it. Nannie knew of my fascination with the mustache cup and repeatedly told me that it would be mine when she died. Jim, however, was adamant that the mustache cup was never to leave the house.

When Nannie died, I took her vintage sewing machine which she had promised me, along with her huge, black leather Bible. Both the Bible and the sewing machine have remained by my bedside in a display table since her death. Having them there makes me feel Nannie close to me and brings fond memories of her. After Nannie's funeral, I walked through the living room and observed the mustache cup still sitting in its home on the mantle. I wanted to take the cup, but Jim's words, "That mustache cup is to never leave this house" echoed in my mind. I walked away in disappointment, as I knew Nannie wanted me to have it. Jim didn't offer the cup to me, and I was well aware of the rage which would erupt if I took it, so I didn't touch it.

When Ruby offered me the mustache cup after Jim's death, I heard Jim's command again. I could not enjoy having it in my home as it would evoke painful memories. He destroyed the pleasure I took from looking at the cup that Nannie wanted me to have. With sadness and regret I told Ruby, "No, I don't want it."

"Don't be so childish, take it," she replied.

But I couldn't. The last time I saw the cup it was sitting on her bureau, broken in several places. If Nannie could have seen it she would have been devastated, as was I. It's hard to believe that a simple antique mustache cup could create such heartache. It wasn't the cup; it was Jim's control—his dominance—that ruined the meaning of the cup for me.

I needed help dealing with my losses when I returned to Labrador City after Jim's death. I had been attending a Survivors of Sexual Abuse Group at the local hospital. One day I was feeling particularly sad and needed to talk, so I instinctively called my counsellor from the survivors' group. She was out of the office but another counsellor was available. Our talk was helpful; I needed to unload some of my grief. I began to realize that I was not only grieving the loss of Jim, but I was also grieving the loss of a father who never was and never would be. It was complicated.

"When it rains, it pours," as the saying goes. While struggling to cope with Jim's death and the fallout from it, a phone call on Christmas Day notified us that Bill's oldest sister, Sandra, just forty-nine years old, had laid down on her bed and passed away from a massive heart attack. It was an extremely difficult time. I desperately wanted to go to the funeral but was just not well enough. Lisa went with Bill while I stayed home with William. I've always regretted that I was unable to attend.

When I attended the inpatient treatment program for families of alcoholics it was recommended that I get counselling for my sexual abuse. This led me to the Survivors of Sexual Abuse Group. I attempted to get the help I needed with my grief from this group, but it wasn't working for me. I wasn't at a point where I was comfortable with others knowing that I was in counselling, although I made no effort to hide my past. I wanted to be in control, and going to counselling meant I wasn't in control. Living and working in a small community where everyone knew me made it challenging to seek the help I knew I desperately needed.

The local United Church minister, Rev. Florence Sanna, offered private counselling in her home, which seemed a perfect fit for me. I went out on a limb and asked her to help me with the grief I was experiencing. In order to heal, I needed to work through the guilt and anger, and, most of all, the many losses in my life that left a huge ball of sadness I couldn't seem to shake. I had much to learn about forgiveness. Rev. Sanna was there to help me understand that forgiveness was for me, and it was a way to release my feelings of resentment toward those who had caused harm to me. I learned that forgiving did not mean I was condoning what was done to me.

I believe that people come into our lives at a time when we need them most. Rev. Florence Sanna was one of those special people. She helped me through many of my most painful childhood memories and helped me understand it was okay to harbour resentment and anger toward my parents—that it was normal to feel guilt for having these feelings. I understood all of this in my head, but my heart couldn't process them without her guidance. My lightbulb moment came when she asked, "Debbie, if you could have chosen your parents, would you have chosen Jim and Ruby?"

Without any hesitation whatsoever, I answered, "No!"

At the time I was seeing Rev. Sanna, I was making a cross-stitch of a little girl picking flowers. The little girl represented me, the loss of a childhood and the pain I felt. A tear fell as I made each stitch. At the top, I stitched, "Please be patient…I'm still growing in God's way." The words came from a church pamphlet that was laying on Rev. Sanna's coffee table. Those words spoke to the little girl within who, as an adult, was still growing and healing. I needed to be patient with myself.

I was in desperate need of validation and needed someone to tell me that what I felt was not in my imagination. I wanted to know that I was understood. Jim and Ruby were incapable of providing validation. They were incapable of understanding my feelings, and they dismissed any concerns I brought forward. When Jim died and Ruby and David put him on a pedestal, both of them belittled me for speaking the truth about my home life. They discounted my experiences as little more than lies.

Rev. Sanna provided validation for me. She allowed me to talk about aspects of my childhood that I tended to minimize, especially the loss of my twin sister, Daphne. I've always felt a connection to her but didn't talk about it because I feared being judged. Rev. Sanna showed me that it was normal to grieve for my sister. After a session with Rev. Sanna in which we talked about Daphne, I had an interesting dream. In the dream, a woman was lying on top of me; I felt a comforting, warm, deep love as we lay together. Upon wakening, at first the dream seemed strange, but I soon realized that it was symbolic of myself and Daphne in Ruby's womb. My mind often brings me back to the peacefulness I experienced during this dream. I believe Daphne is with me and has been throughout my life. I look forward to meeting her again in the next realm.

When I gave myself permission to talk about Daphne, I felt more comfort with it. I was always troubled that she was buried in an unmarked grave in a corner of the Anglican cemetery in Burnside because she wasn't baptized in the Anglican Church, so I decided it was time to right this wrong. I ordered a child's headstone for Daphne and tried to figure out how to place it now that the cemetery was full to capacity. I was concerned that I if asked for the go-ahead to place the headstone I would be denied. Upon the advice of a wise Anglican authority, I didn't seek permission, I just had the headstone placed beside Nannie's headstone. Giving Daphne the recognition she deserved helped bring closure for me.

Ruby and I weren't on good terms then, and I didn't tell her what I was doing. I didn't want anyone to object, so I kept it to myself. Ruby didn't mention seeing the headstone for a long time, but to my disbelief, she was very pleased with the action I had taken. For a brief moment, it felt as though her and I had a connection. Although she didn't say so, I believe it helped to bring closure for her as well.

Lisa

There are many funny stories that we now reminisce about from Lisa's childhood. One story that we often retell is about Lisa taking a bag of dirty kitty litter off the back step of our house on her way to school in grade two. She had left the house when I realized her lunch was still on the kitchen table. I hurried to catch her before she went too far down the street.

"Lisa, come back. You forgot your lunch!" I called.

Lifting up a plastic bag to show me, she called out, "I've got my lunch."

"Where did you get the bag?"

"I took it off the top of the barbeque," she replied.

Through bursts of laughter I said, "Lisa, that's the dirty kitty litter. Here's your lunch."

She ran back so we could exchange bags. I'm laughing out loud as I write this story. To this day none of us can figure out why she took the very heavy bag of dirty kitty litter off the top of the barbeque and thought it was her lunch. I had never put her lunch outside for her to claim on the way to school. It's an extremely funny puzzle that I just couldn't resist sharing.

Just when you think life is beginning to run smoothly, something interrupts the flow. I didn't expect to have difficulties raising my children because I was parenting the opposite way I had learned from my parents. Surely this meant my children would grow up without giving us issues. Oh boy, was I wrong on that one! Once they hit the teen years everything changed.

Uncharacteristically, and more so out of curiosity, I saw a psychic. I was in disbelief when he told me so many things regarding my life that were factual.

"Your daughter is an asshole magnet," he said.

I asked him to repeat himself several times, as I had never heard the term before. His description of Lisa couldn't have been more accurate.

Lisa's teenage years were challenging. She had difficulty fitting in with her peers, she was bullied at school and not accepted for who she was. Try as she might, she just couldn't find a place where she belonged, so she found friends like herself who also didn't fit the norm.

Lisa suffered with what we first thought were growing pains in her legs, as well as severe stomach pain in her younger years and was diagnosed with juvenile arthritis. I'll forever remember the day she showed me that her baby fingers wouldn't straighten out. All of her joints were tender and her ligaments were shrinking, causing her limbs to bend. Her illness was, and still is, a mystery. The pediatrician prescribed Naprosyn E which, among other side effects, caused her hair to fall out.

Lisa educated herself about her illness because she thought it would be helpful to tell others in school about it, but this backfired on her. Instead of being accepted with understanding, the kids made fun of her. Try as she might, she couldn't win, so her attitude changed. She became quiet, and her once outgoing personally was replaced with low self-esteem, which attracted the bullies.

Lisa's home life was structured. We had weekly family meetings, ate supper together, enforced a curfew and gave her chores and responsibilities. She gravitated toward friends whose home life was different from hers. They had no rules and could come and go as they pleased with no consequences. Lisa bristled against our rules. No one in our family remembers exactly what the issue was, but she decided to leave home and stay with a friend. I was devastated! I strived to be a good parent, the opposite of what I grew up with. When Lisa left home, although her frustration with us was short lived, I felt like a failure. It was as if she had stuck a knife through my heart. I was helpless.

Bill was the rational parent, assuring me that Lisa would come to her senses and return home. She did, and all was well. She guarantees me that it was just "teenage stuff." Since we can't remember what Lisa was concerned about, I guess it was just a passing moment in a teenage girl's life where she felt the need to rebel.

Lisa's first crush was on a boy she met while we were visiting with her cousin in Rose Blanche, Newfoundland. They kept in touch after we returned to Labrador City. There were no phone plans in the 1990s, you paid by the minute. I knew she was talking to him because I made her hang up late at night numerous times. When I got my $500+ phone bill, I put a stop to the conversations and made her repay the money from her allowance.

Lisa was sneaky as a teenager, but she usually got caught. We occasionally let her use our snowmobile. On an evening that Bill and I were attending an event where we wouldn't be readily available if she needed us, we told her that she wasn't to touch the snowmobile. Being a typical rebellious teenager, Lisa decided she would take the snowmobile and be home before we knew anything about it. Unfortunately for her, the machine broke down on the lake, and she had to call her Uncle Bert to tow it home.

I tried to respect Lisa's privacy as much as a parent can, but as I mentioned she usually got caught. For whatever reason we haven't been able to understand, Lisa left her diary open on my bureau. Of course, when I saw the open pages I read them and learned she had experimented with alcohol.

When Lisa started dating, her first boyfriend, Brad, seemed fine. She brought him to meet us, and he ate with us at our home. As time went on we realized Lisa was changing. She was no longer the outgoing, bubbly, fun-loving, caring, self-confident girl we had grown to love. Her whole life revolved around him, and her girlfriends disappeared. He demanded her undivided attention. It seemed the more Bill and I tried to help her understand that this was an unhealthy relationship, the more she gravitated toward him.

We became extremely concerned after we witnessed an outburst of Brad's anger. Bill was cooking ribs for supper and had to leave to pick me up from work. He asked Lisa to watch the ribs in the oven to make sure they didn't burn. Upon checking the ribs when he got home, Bill found them burnt, so he questioned Lisa. Brad rushed into the kitchen yelling, "Leave Lisa the fuck alone. You're always fucking picking on her!" Bill and I were shocked; we couldn't believe what we were witnessing. Bill told him to leave and that he wasn't welcome back in our home.

As a counsellor I saw the red flags, and I was determined not to give up. I made every effort to keep the lines of communication open with

Lisa. I insisted that she watch videos and read literature about abusive relationships, and I reached out to other counsellors who worked at the local women's shelter to introduce Lisa to them.

It felt like we were in a tug of war and Brad was winning, but I wasn't prepared to give up that easily. School was over and we were going on vacation to PEI and Newfoundland. Lisa was adamant that she was not going with us and wanted to stay with Brad's parents. Bill and I would not back down. We knew we had to get Lisa away from Labrador City and Brad. We hoped that the distance would help Lisa break free of the control he had over her, and it worked!

When we arrived in Newfoundland, Lisa, who had just gotten her license, was delighted to take our vehicle and meet new friends. We were eager to give her freedom to be herself, and we saw a glimpse of the beautiful girl she was until Brad trapped her into a relationship in which his power and control made her a victim of dating abuse. I believe she would not have been able to set herself free if we hadn't taken her away from him.

Brad's grip on Lisa wasn't completely gone; he kept in touch with her. She went back to high school in September, and he went to college in Goose Bay. We hoped the distance would put her on the road to freedom from him, and she even started dating again. Brad learned of her new relationship and decided to hitchhike from Goose Bay to Labrador City to confront Marty, Lisa's new boyfriend. Brad encountered Marty in the school parking lot where they had a physical altercation. The police were called, and Brad was charged with assault. Lisa was home for lunch at the time, and the guidance counsellor called to say she should stay home, as they were concerned for her safety. Lisa, however, insisted on going back to school. For her protection, she waited in the guidance counsellor's office, where he invited her to colour dating violence posters.

These events resulted in a restraining order being placed on Brad by the police. He was to have no contact with Lisa or Marty, but a piece of paper meant nothing to Brad, and he remained in contact with Lisa. Bill and I were concerned for her safety, but despite our vigilance, it took some time for Lisa to break away entirely from Brad.

The incident when Brad assaulted Marty coincided with a call from the principal at William's school saying he was suspended for the day.

Apparently, students weren't permitted to leave school during lunch break but William had other plans. When he was caught leaving he refused to come back and cursed at the teacher.

While all this was happening Bill was working nightshift. Between the calls from school and the police, he was unable to get any sleep. I was attending a conference in St. John's, so he was on his own. And thus began the trials and tribulations of raising two teenagers. I'll talk more about our son later.

Gradually, Lisa began to understand the dynamics of being in an abusive relationship. The guidance counsellor at school and counsellors from the women's shelter called on Lisa to talk with other young women who were also in abusive relationships. Lisa assisted representatives from the shelter when they gave presentations about dating violence. These opportunities were empowering for Lisa and helped her gain back her self-esteem.

When Lisa turned sixteen we insisted she look for work because we wanted her to learn responsibility. She found a waitressing job and worked on weekends. She bought her own clothes and personal items and put gas in the car. Prior to getting a job, Lisa would never have dreamed of shopping at a thrift store but soon realized she could have inexpensive and quality clothes. While Lisa had to work, her friends were just hanging around. They told her we were mean parents. In their minds, since Bill and I both had good jobs and made decent money, Lisa shouldn't have to work. Lisa has reassured us that she's thankful we made her go to work.

After high school graduation, Lisa entered the Culinary Arts Program at Holland College in Prince Edward Island. She returned to Labrador City where she worked various jobs in the food services industry. She was independent, got her own apartment, often worked two jobs and was self-sufficient.

Lisa became interested in starting her own wedding decorating business, and Bill had taken an early retirement from the Iron Ore Company of Canada so he became her right-hand man. Eventually, Lisa's business evolved into a family business known as Lisa's Decorations and Creations. Lisa and Bill worked together to decorate for weddings and community events, and they catered weddings and Christmas parties. Lisa DJ'd and was in great demand, so we decided to expand the business to include the Labrador City Arena Canteen. It truly was a family business. I did the accounting and everyone chipped in when they could to help with the decorating, catering and canteen.

Lisa had a few relationships in her early twenties, as most young people do, but nothing serious. Then she met Bram. They dated for a few years and then got married. Lisa and Bram dreamed of starting a family.

After a few years of trying to conceive, Lisa was advised that in vitro fertilization (IVF) would be her best option, so they went to Calgary for the procedure. Sadly, the doctors botched the procedure and almost took my daughter's life. In the process of transferring her eggs they clipped her bladder and ovary. This led to a massive infection behind her uterus and bowels. During the evening following the IVF procedure, Lisa suffered excruciating pain, and Bram was terrified. He immediately called 911, and they went by ambulance to the hospital where she was examined. Although she was still unwell, she was advised that she was okay to leave Calgary and return to Labrador, so they released her from hospital. Lisa became extremely ill during the flight, was taken off the plane in Toronto and rushed by ambulance to the nearest hospital. Again, although her health was deteriorating, she was released and told it was okay to fly back to Labrador City.

Lisa's health continued to deteriorate when she arrived home. When I went to check on her, I had to call the ambulance. Bram accompanied her on the air ambulance to the Health Sciences Centre in St. John's. I flew to St. John's the following day, and William also took time off work and flew out to be with his sister. Bill wanted to be there but someone had to care for Lisa and William's pets, so he volunteered.

I rented an apartment and a car while we were in St. John's, and one of us stayed with Lisa at all times. Bram bought an air mattress to sleep on beside her bed. Watching my daughter so seriously ill was heartbreaking and terrifying. I made every effort to be brave for her and Bram, but inside I was terrified.

The day finally came when she was told she had miscarried her twins. Knowing this was their last chance to have a family, we were all devastated. Lisa and Bram's dreams were crushed, and watching their disappointment was unbearably painful. My memory of my beautiful daughter in the hospital bed looking frail, weak and lost is something that will never leave me. My heart goes out to any woman and her family who have to go through such a traumatic experience.

Lisa and Bram have since moved to the west coast of Newfoundland where they are both working. They live a quiet, peaceful and happy life in the country with their bulldog, Reggie, and Boston terrier, Margo. To my absolute delight they have just applied to become foster parents. I only wish there had been a "Lisa and Bram" for me when I was a troubled teen. They will make a huge impact on the lives of the children who come into their care.

The relationship I have with Lisa today is better than I ever could have imagined. I've always told her, "If there were rows and rows of daughters to choose from, I'd always choose you!" When Lisa got married she asked me to be her maid of honour. I was taken aback as I had never heard of such a thing. I asked her why she wanted me to do it and her answer warms my heart to this day: "You're my best friend, Mom."

Lisa and Bram live just an hour from us, and we see them often. Bram is our second "son" who fit into our family from day one. They have blessed our family, and I am forever grateful to have a close and caring bond with them.

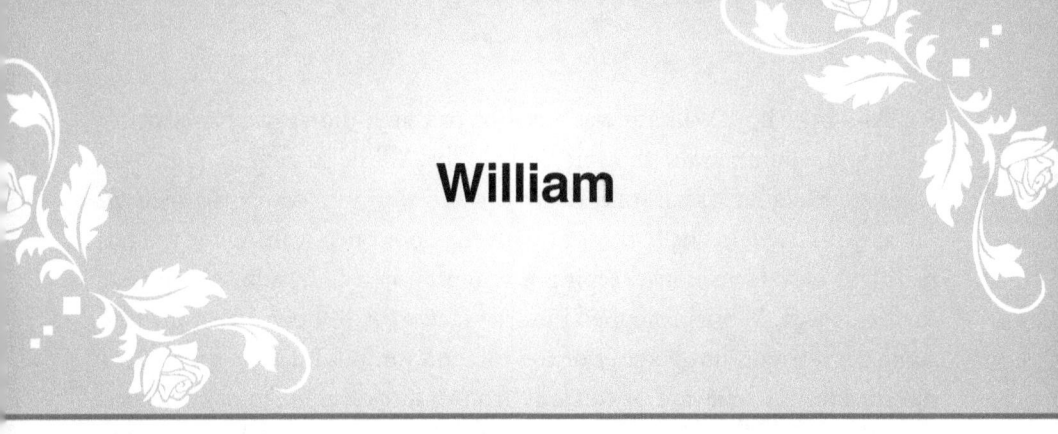

William

William was a force to be reckoned with when he was little. He threw temper tantrums when he didn't get his own way. On one occasion Bill had to walk away from him in an aisle at Toys "R" Us until a tantrum ended. There was no reasoning with him when the mood hit; he screamed, cried and kicked until he tired himself out.

We still tease William about the "lines" in his socks. As a child he became extremely frustrated when the seam in his socks didn't fit exactly right across his foot. We would all breathe a sigh of relief when he got his socks on without an issue.

William was a strong-willed, independent child; he wanted to do it his way, and he tested us. I recall walking to a neighbour's house with him in the winter when there was a lot of snow and ice on her steps. I tried to hold his hand but, lo and behold, he refused, let go of my hand and fell. He hit his chin on the concrete step, which required a trip to the hospital and stitches.

Not long after I started working full time and studying, I decided to have someone do the housecleaning, and I found a wonderful lady named Paulette. Her and I had many great chats when she came to clean, and we became the best of friends. After one time when Paulette had finished cleaning, she grinned and said to me, "Debbie, I don't think William likes me touching the stuff in his bedroom."

"No, he probably doesn't. Why?" I replied.

"He has a bicycle chain lock wrapped around his toys," she said.

When we questioned William about this he bluntly said he didn't want his toys moved. Even at a very young age William liked order. We have had lots of laughs over the years about William's bike lock.

As a little boy, William was terrified of water, didn't want to learn to swim and wouldn't take showers, only baths. While staying in a hotel on vacation when he was around five, we convinced him to try the Jacuzzi. He and Bill were in the bathroom with the door open waiting for the tub to fill. A lady from housekeeping was replacing a lightbulb just outside the bathroom. William stepped into the Jacuzzi as Bill turned on the jets, so he got a fright, jumped out of the tub and ran out into the room buttnaked. He was unaware of the lady from housekeeping, so as he leaped onto the bed and saw her, without hesitation, he nearly flew back into the bathroom. It was the most comical sight. I've never seen him move so fast, so much so that I'm doubtful the lady even realized what was happening. It's a story that our family has recalled over and over, and it always evokes belly laughter.

The fact that William has a learning disability contributed to his dislike for school. He is very smart but, like his dad, has difficulty with the written aspect of learning. Methods of teaching just didn't fit the style of learning which could have been beneficial to William's education. Thus, from an early age, he developed a dislike for school and, like his sister, gravitated to others like him.

When Bill went to school in the 1970s he was considered lazy or unintelligent. I didn't grasp that William was struggling until I went to parent-teacher interviews in grade one. His teacher explained that he was trying really hard but truly had trouble understanding certain areas of the curriculum.

Our family has come to realize that "book" learning is not all that it's cracked up to be. When my children went to school there was a push toward university. Thankfully, times are changing and trades are given more of the acceptance and importance they deserve. One job is as important as the next. Every person can contribute, whether it is with their brains or brawn.

Most days I would receive a call from the office asking if it was okay for William to leave school. We lived a couple minutes within walking distance to his high school, and he told me he needed to come home to use the washroom. We laugh now when I ask him if he needs to come home from work to use the washroom.

Skipping school became the norm for William, and it was a struggle to get him up in the morning. On the vast majority of school days, when I returned home from work, there was a voice message on my phone saying, "A student from your home was absent from school today."

We made every effort to have a structured home life for William. He resisted, but we persisted. Every Friday after supper was family meeting time. He was annoyed because his friends would be waiting outside for him but would leave when he didn't come out. It was important to keep the lines of communication open with both of our children, and though it was challenging, I know we did the right thing by not giving in. Through all the struggles, we managed to raise two responsible children and we have maintained a family bond that has not wavered.

William's first brush with the law came when he was just twelve years old. His friend, who was already known to police, decided to break into a house where he knew there was money. William and another friend waited outside while he went in and stole the money, and William was charged with break and enter. He was placed on house arrest and ordered to do community service, repay the money and write an apology letter.

William's next encounter with the police was for drinking underage. Not long after this charge, the police knocked on our door advising us that they suspected William had possession of marijuana. There was no evidence, but he was charged anyway. I have no problem with justice being served if one is guilty, but it is concerning when there is no evidence. We hired a lawyer to represent William on the possession charge, and the judge threw out the case. Before doing so, however, he gave William a stern lecture.

"If I ever see you back in my courtroom, I will have you sent to a group home," he said.

Upon hearing this, I got my back up really fast.

"Over my dead body will they ever send you to a group home!" I said to William.

I was serious. I would be on the tarmac in front of the airplane if they ever tried to take William away from me. I know all too well what happens when a child is put in "care," and there was no way they would ever take my son. I am a fighter, and this is one fight I would not back down from. Fortunately, that was the end of William's legal issues while he was a juvenile.

With William out of school during the summer months, it was not easy to keep track of his whereabouts. I recall waking up in the wee hours of the morning and discovering that he wasn't home. I was distraught and nervously waited at the kitchen table until he showed up. We had a conversation in which I tried to help him understand that we needed to know where he was and that he was safe. After some sincere negotiations, we agreed that if he was going to "sneak out" he would write me a note, saying what time he was leaving and where he was going. His friends couldn't believe that he was permitted to "sneak out." It was not an ideal situation, but I knew I couldn't lock him in his room. What was a parent to do? He says it took the fun out of it for him.

William started working with Bessey's Movers when he was just thirteen. When he turned sixteen he was hired to stock shelves and bag and carry out groceries at the local Co-Op.

William's teenage years were typical of many young people; partying, drinking and using drugs were common. I was concerned but tried to chalk it up to typical experimentation. Although the struggle was real for William, he did graduate from high school. Unsure of what he wanted to do, he headed to Alberta. While on this adventure he experienced a lot of trauma, such as being in a bar while there was a shooting. After a couple of months, and to my relief, he returned to Labrador City where he worked as a labourer with contractors.

It became more and more obvious that William had a drinking problem. It was devastating to watch my son spiral down to a place where, try as I might, I could not reach him. A part of me was in denial, and I didn't want to believe that this was happening to my child. As addicts do, he minimized his drinking and drug use when I confronted him. I wondered when he would hit his bottom. Being a parent of an alcoholic child left me feeling helpless. One of my greatest fears was that he would kill himself or someone else when he was drinking. He had many close calls, two impaired drinking charges and numerous accidents.

Through all of the trauma I watched William experience as an addict, the most terrifying moment was the phone call I received from my friend, Cynt. I could hear the concern in her voice as she asked, "Is William okay?"

"Why? What are you talking about? He's at work," I said.

She said maybe she misunderstood but she heard he went through the ice on a snowmobile. I immediately called William, and I instinctively knew from the tone of his voice that something was wrong. He sounded distant, and it was difficult to get answers from him. Eventually I came to understand he had been drinking, and he drove his snowmobile, with a friend on behind him, for a spin on the lake. It was a bitterly cold night of -50°C. While speeding across the lake, unable to see what was ahead, he suddenly plunged into the frigid water. Somehow he managed to swim to shore while helping to save his friend from drowning. He was aware they were at the edge of the lake close to Wabush Mines, and he knew the area because he had worked in the mine. He and his friend managed to crawl and drag themselves through the snow and ice to a work shack in the area. Dripping wet and close to hypothermia, they survived the ordeal by staying in the shack and out of the elements until one of their cellphones dried out enough to make a call for help.

I cringe as I write about this terrifying episode and realize that we could have lost our son. The residual effects of this near-death experience still remain with William.

My years of Al-Anon taught me well, and I knew I should not enable William. It was a struggle because I love my son and would do anything to remove his pain, so I ended up being an enabler even against my better judgement. While he was still living at home I called him to go to work. Many mornings I could smell alcohol when I opened his room door. He usually didn't want to get up because he had been out drinking most of the night. However, because I so desperately wanted him to be responsible and successful, I refused to let him fail. Hindsight is 20/20, as the saying goes. Despite all my efforts to push William to at least keep a job, he was fired (from a job I helped him get) for being at work under the influence.

Never in my wildest dreams did I think my child would be an alcoholic. How could this be happening? I grew up in an alcoholic home and married an alcoholic, now I was living the nightmare of having an alcoholic child. I questioned our parenting. Could we have done something to make him choose this path? He has assured me that it was not because of anything we did or did not do. I did many things to enable William's addiction to progress although I was totally aware that I shouldn't.

I was determined, even if it took me to my last breath, to stick by our son and love him unconditionally. I knew it was crucial for us to be there for him when he fell and needed a soft place to land. I tried to, as the saying goes in Al-Anon, "Let Go and Let God."

Sometimes I let it go, and other times I took it back.

I spent too many sleepless nights worrying about William and even followed his cell phone with an app (unbeknownst to him, of course). I justified it in my mind because I knew he was reckless when he used drugs or drank.

Despite his addiction, William had the drive to get his Heavy Equipment Operator Certificate from the College of the North Atlantic, was hired at Wabush Mines and made a very good living.

William was in a relationship but it was quite clear that it was unhealthy. Against our advice, he bought a house with her. Eventually, the relationship ended and bills weren't being paid. One day I watched his truck (and our $5,000 collateral) get towed away and repossessed. The writing was on the wall; bankruptcy was inevitable. Bill and I made every effort to bail William out, sinking our own money into a situation that was doomed for failure.

Realizing that our son would soon be homeless, we tried to find a way to help (as we always did). Coincidentally, while on our morning walk, Bill and I came across a trailer for sale privately. It was too good a deal to pass up so we bought it as a rental property. In the back of my mind, I knew it would eventually be a home for William. True to my intuition, the ink was barely dry on the deed when William's house was repossessed, so he moved into the trailer. As he was still in active alcoholism and drug addiction, to ensure he paid rent, I had him put my name on his bank account.

William started dating Lynn in 2010. She was fresh out of a relationship with Lee, who made our family's lives a living hell from the beginning.

One time when William and Lynn went camping, William's yellow Lab, Samps, was left at home overnight. Lisa went to check on Samps in the morning. To her shock, the porch door was kicked in and Samps lay trembling on the kitchen floor. Ordinarily, Samps would have ran away when he saw the opportunity of an open door. She immediately called the police and her father. Shortly after Bill and the police arrived, to everyone's surprise, Lee and his father showed up. Lee confessed that he was the culprit, which came as no surprise as he had an altercation with Lynn and William the previous night.

Lee was charged, pled guilty and was convicted of mischief relating to property damage, failure to comply with a condition of undertaking, assault, and uttering threats to cause death or bodily harm. He was ordered to pay me for the replacement of the door he destroyed and to not contact or communicate with William, Lisa, Bill or myself.

This event had been extremely traumatic for our family, so prior to Lee's court appearance I made contact with the provincial Victim Services Department. We lived in fear of what Lee's next move would be and didn't feel safe in our own homes, so I wrote a Victim Impact Statement for Lee's court hearing. I felt it was important for the court to understand how Lee's violent behaviour affected us.

It didn't help. The next six years were a living nightmare for our family. I felt defeated each time I called the police because there was never enough evidence to convict Lee. Our family knew, however, that he was using tactics to instill fear in us, especially William. There were incidents of eggs thrown at William's window, and he drove by our home screeching his tires and flipping his middle finger at us.

Lynn and Lee have a beautiful daughter who was ten months old when William started dating Lynn. Their daughter became a big part of our family from the very beginning. We love her, as she does us, and this infuriated Lee. I once received a phone call from him in which he said, "If you buy stuff for my daughter it'll be a waste of your money because I'll throw it all out. I don't want you around her. You better respect what I'm telling you. If you don't, there will be trouble. I'll guarantee you, I'll make things miserable for everyone. Your son is a fucking loser, alcoholic. You can help everyone else, but you can't help him."

I refused to let Lee's threats intimidate me. Lynn was perfectly fine with her daughter spending time with our family and, with her permission, we continued to do so. Despite Lee's interferences, William and Lynn remained in a relationship.

I agonized for a long time over writing about this situation with Lee because I feared it would put a strain on the great relationship I have with him and his family today. In the end, however, I knew I couldn't exclude it from my book because it was a time in my life that was extremely traumatic. Lee has apologized for his behaviour. Apologies are useless, in my opinion, unless one changes their behaviour. In this case, I see a changed man. I feel extremely comfortable talking to Lee. I have no bitterness toward him, and I have forgiven him.

A few years ago Lee was at a New Year's Eve celebration where I was, and it was a sincere pleasure to be in his company. I have an excellent relationship with his mom. I don't believe that sharing this part of my life will affect the understanding Lee, his family and I have of each other; good relationships endure. I enjoy having opportunities to show that people can change and hurts can be mended, as is the case with Lee and me.

William's drinking and drug use escalated through all of this turmoil, and I grew more and more concerned for his well-being. As difficult as it was, I tried to remain hopeful and positive.

A relaxing vacation in New York City with Josephine quickly turned into a nightmare when I began receiving phone calls from William in the wee hours of the morning. Him and Lynn were on a trip to Cuba for a friend's wedding. William had gotten drunk and they had fight. During the flight to Cuba William suffered an alcoholic seizure and was hauled from his seat by passengers, causing a rotator cuff injury. The airline questioned whether they would allow him on a return flight to Canada. While all of this was being relayed to me by William, I wanted to support him but my helplessness increased by the fact that he was in another country. It was comforting to have Josephine's empathetic ear throughout this ordeal. Eventually the mess was sorted out and William returned home. This is just another example of the stress I faced with an alcoholic son. It was difficult to let my guard down and relax as I never knew what was around the corner. My body was constantly in the fight/flight/freeze response.

On a weekend in the summer of 2010 while we were camping, Bill and I went for an early morning walk. We noticed a car in the woods that was wedged upon a rock. As we got closer we realized it was William's car. Our hearts sank; we were terrified to learn what had happened to William. Was he alive? Was he hurt? Did he injure someone? Did he kill someone?

We discovered that William had been drinking, gotten into a fight with Lynn and stormed off in his car. He was driving through trails in the woods, drove onto a rock in the path and got the car stuck. A passerby phoned the police, and William was charged with DUI.

This may have been the bottom we were waiting for. William finally admitted he had an addiction and needed help. He started going for counselling at the local mental health department. Eventually, he and his counsellor agreed that he required inpatient treatment, so he attended the Humberwood Treatment Centre in Corner Brook, NL.

I was involved with the Labrador West Chapter of Mothers Against Drunk Driving (MADD). Coincidentally, while William was in treatment, the local MADD chapter hosted a public forum on impaired driving. I was part of a panel of people who spoke about the issue from various perspectives. The event was broadcast on the CBC NL *Here and Now* supper hour news. With William's permission, I laid bare what it was like to have an alcoholic son. It was a "no-holds-barred" perspective—raw and revealing from beginning to end. William had informed staff and patients at Humberwood about the forum, so they gathered around the TV to watch it. William said it was "powerful." It was a relief to speak openly about the struggles of raising and living with an alcoholic child.

Our family and friends were extremely proud of William. Conquering an addiction is one of the hardest things a person can face in life. William had taken the first step in admitting he had an addiction and needed help. He was finally out of denial and on the road to recovery, which meant we could all sleep a little easier at night.

William was home from Humberwood for only a couple of months when he relapsed, which is a normal part of recovery. As a counsellor, I was more than aware of this fact, but that didn't make it less difficult to deal with. However, it was somewhat easier to talk to William about his addiction this time around. He no longer refused to admit he had a problem, and he acknowledged he needed more help to overcome his addiction. He also confessed that he knew he would have another DUI if he didn't get sober. He decided to go back to see his counsellor at the mental health department and was made a candidate to attend a longer, more intense addiction treatment program at the Homewood Treatment Facility in Guelph, ON.

Lisa and William are very close siblings who worship the ground the other walks on. Lisa was determined to literally wash away all the bad memories William had in his home, so she cleaned and painted his place throughout, hung treasured pictures on the walls, redecorated and rearranged while he was in rehab. Lisa instinctively knew the makeover would help ease the burden of returning to a place where so much of William's life had been in turmoil. When William completed the program and returned home, we were all eager to see his reaction to his sister's hard work. He was in shock. He sat on the floor in the kitchen and wept.

"I can't believe it! I don't know what to say!" he said through the tears. "I was dreading coming in here to face the bad memories."

A ton of weight was lifted from my shoulders when William started his recovery journey after Homewood. When one's life is touched by addiction, there's always a twinge of fear that the addict will be pulled back into their addiction, but I fought to push that fear away in order to enjoy the excitement of watching our son make positive changes in his life.

Spiralling Down

Once in 2010 and again in 2011, I had become ill and was put off work for a month each time, but I pushed myself to return to work because my career was very important to me. I worked hard to get where I was, and I desperately wanted to get back there. In hindsight, I realize that a mental illness was brewing.

February 2, 2012, was the day I lost the battle with the beast. I fought it for years and years, but the more I fought, the bigger and hungrier it grew. It became too powerful for me to fight any longer. I cried like a baby as I admitted defeat.

I was on my way back to work after lunch when I realized I could not make it through the remainder of the day. As I drove the highway I contemplated how I could drive my truck off the road and kill myself. I was trying to figure a way out, but I was afraid I wouldn't die if I drove the truck off the road. I was desperate for a way out of my misery.

As I walked into my office, I called out to Pam and Josephine and collapsed in the fetal position.

"I can't do this anymore!" I said through my sobbing.

I managed to pull myself together with the help of my faithful co-workers/friends, and I made an appointment with my doctor for the following morning. I left that office, never to return to work again.

I was fortunate to have one of the best doctors in the province, Dr. Tom Costello, winner of the 2019 Newfoundland & Labrador Family Doctor Award. He was compassionate and understanding and took me off work indefinitely.

I had not been feeling well, mentally, for a long time. I easily became overwhelmed and had great difficulty concentrating. Things I had normally thrived on were becoming more and more difficult to do. Even giving a workshop took every ounce of effort I had. The stress of working in an extremely unhealthy environment was taking its toll on me. I would cry to Bill at night that I didn't know how much longer I could carry on because I felt my life crumbling around me.

After almost twenty years of working independently and with superiors who went above and beyond to support my work, I was taken off guard when a couple of new individuals came on the scene. As it is with large companies, management can change quite often. There were a lot of changes within the organization, particularly new management from outside of the isolated towns of Labrador City and Wabush, and we saw many new people on the scene who brought their own ideas and practices which were different from what was common in the company.

Although I kept telling myself it was my imagination, I experienced bullying and harassment in an underhanded way. I sat in disbelief as a new boss walked into my office and, without saying a word or asking a question, examined every framed certificate on the wall. Because I want to see the best in people, I told myself she was interested in my education. However, since I'd learned to read my gut, I knew she had an ulterior motive.

This new boss said I couldn't continue my employment without my own liability insurance. This was a surprise to me since I worked for a private company who carried their own insurance and I would automatically be covered in case I was sued. Not being one to back down, I made phone calls and wrote emails until I got the answer I was looking for. I was not required to carry my own liability insurance, and I was protected by my employer's insurance.

People questioning my credentials came next. I was required to prove that I was qualified to do my job. After helping people for over twenty years as a counsellor, I was not impressed (to say the least) with all the scrutiny from the new management. Quite frankly, I was offended. However, as I've had to do before, I gathered my education documentation together with my professional designations and complied with the request. After a lengthy wait and much questioning, I was deemed qualified.

The harassment became so stressful I had no choice but to file a complaint with the Human Resources Department, and an external investigator was brought in. Other employees, including a high-profile individual, had shared their stories of harassment with me, so I knew I wasn't alone. However, when the investigation was over I stood alone because no one came forward to share their stories for fear of reprisal.

Despite my disappointment, I wouldn't do it any differently. I had to stand up and say that this individual's behaviour was unacceptable. I didn't have any further issues with the perpetrator after the investigation and didn't hear of additional concerns from employees. Although it was an extremely overwhelming situation, one I wouldn't wish on another person, I hope that standing up for my rights made a difference in others' lives. Everything I had worked so hard to achieve was being questioned and, as difficult as the situation was, I felt empowered!

Next, I was told to share personal information about my clients with a newly created department. From day one, I prided myself on ensuring that all information shared with me by employees and their families was confidential, except when required to report by law (as in a case of suspected child abuse or neglect). I was adamant that I would not share personal information with others just because they were in the same department. I pushed my concern up the ladder and wouldn't back down until I was satisfied that they dropped the matter. Eventually, my determination paid off, and they finally listened to me.

The challenges didn't stop there.

Certain individuals then tried to undermine and intimidate me. They questioned my role in the organization and accused me of "crossing the line." I found myself excluded from important decisions regarding the EFAP and discovered that proven processes I had been involved in were unilaterally changed. I wasn't invited to important meetings or copied on relevant emails. I could go on, but I think you get the picture.

I had a gut feeling that something wasn't right when I had a visit from a person in upper management who was new to the organization. She questioned everything about my role and appeared to be supportive. However, it was she who accused me of "crossing the line." In my role of mediating harassment in the workplace I had been a mediator in a serious case between two co-workers and, as was the practice, I had made a recommendation to HR regarding the situation. When I received an email with her allegation against me I was shocked and couldn't understand her concern.

I spoke to my boss about the situation and asked for a meeting to get clarification. Every time the meeting was scheduled there was a reason why she had to cancel, so I didn't know what I should or shouldn't do in my role. The career I had so cherished was changing, and I felt helpless. I was being micromanaged, and I don't do well in this type of environment.

Although there was a lot on my plate and I was mentally and physically exhausted, I constantly forced myself to get things done and continued to push for a meeting to resolve my concern about the accusation of "crossing the line" at work. Finally, I received notification that a meeting was planned for April 5. At the last minute, I was informed I could not attend this meeting because of my illness unless I received medical clearance from my doctor. I was distraught, as this information came at the closing of the work day on April 4. Determined to get to the bottom of this, I reached out to my counsellor, Annette, who agreed to accompany me to the meeting.

I will forever be grateful that I did not attend this meeting alone. How could I have possibly known what was in store? We were met at the door of the building and directed to an office in the basement. When I knocked on the door, to my astonishment, a representative from Human Resources opened the door. I literally stepped back and almost knocked Annette down. I knew that something wasn't right about this scene.

As I stepped into the room I realized that the person who had accused me of "crossing the line" was not there. I was not prepared for what came next. I was advised that the internal EFAP office was being replaced with an external EFAP provider and that a psychologist was available in the next room if I needed to talk to someone. Having Annette with me was one of the best decisions we could have made because I'm not sure how I would have gotten through the meeting without her. I knew this meeting meant the end of my career with this company. I was given a list of positions I could apply for and told that a representative from HR would be in contact with me.

My co-workers, Pam and Josephine, were then called in, without warning, and advised that their services were no longer required. The locks were changed on the office doors, our computer passwords and voicemail messages were changed, and then it got worse. Pam, Josephine and I were told to meet an HR representative at the EFAP office the following Monday morning so we could retrieve our personal belongings.

I felt numb as we walked into that office for the last time. Watching my husband take my certificates off the wall was overwhelming; it was as if someone died. Everything I had worked so hard to achieve was being ripped away. Over twenty years of pouring my heart and soul into a dream was disappearing. Something that worked so well and helped hundreds of people was, in someone's opinion, no longer needed.

Little did this company know that employees would not be happy with their decision to outsource a program that had been a staple in the lives of so many. It didn't sit well with employees and their families that they would now have to call a 1-800 number for counselling. There would be no more face-to-face counselling or other services provided by the program, such as assistance filing for death benefits. Employees were upset with the way the whole situation unfolded. As my co-worker, Josephine, bluntly said in a letter to the editor of the local newspaper, "We were made to feel like common criminals—guilty of what?"

My shock wasn't over yet. I received phone calls from clients who were concerned that the company had access to their files. I alleviated their fears by re-emphasizing that there were no files. I had given my word when I started the program that there would be no records of people who came to see me. Everything I knew and learned from an individual was in my head, not on paper.

The new management did not consult with me, and they made assumptions about the way the program was run, including that there were personal files in the EFAP office. It infuriated me that these people could walk in and, without any consideration whatsoever, potentially destroy the credibility I prided myself on. How dare they make me look like a liar!

To add insult to injury, an interview in the local newspaper with the vice president of human resources said, "The company is maintaining confidentiality with employee files by hiring an independent company specialized with organizing and reducing the risks associated with information protection. The company doesn't want to be in the business of handling these records. We want them to be at arm's length; they're not ours. Employees who wish to obtain their file can do so by request, by signing a release form and picking it up. The independent company can also be the custodian of the files, or if a new counsellor has been found the client can release the files to them."

The inevitable request for the files came. In the midst of all this turmoil, I was not getting the answers I was promised in respect to my future. As I was all too familiar with the processes, I knew I was under investigation, as I was repeatedly asked where the files were. All of this stress was making me sicker. My husband watched on as this company brought me to one of the lowest points I have ever been. He wanted me to sign away any rights I had to compensation. Despite becoming more ill, I was determined to fight, as I am a fighter, and there was still a little part of me that was determined not to back down. I made an appointment with a lawyer who suggested I tell management I would give them answers regarding the files only after they gave me answers, in writing, with respect to my options.

Bill accompanied me to a meeting with HR representatives, where I was able to speak my truth and express how I felt. I told them the way I had been treated by the people in management regarding the closure of the EFAP office was a good example of how not to treat employees, and that I was hurt and deserved better.

Eventually, I received a summary of my options in writing should I be cleared to return to work from my medical leave. This meant I had to produce the files from the EFAP office. I was really taken back when I was asked if I had ever been back to the office since the time I had cleared out my personal effects. If yes, for what purpose? When I was called into the meeting on April 5 and told the EFAP office was being closed, I was advised the locks on the office doors were being changed, so did management think I broke into the second-floor office? I was insulted and hurt by this question.

I explained that, from the onset of the program, employees and their family members were assured of anonymity and confidentiality. There were no files. I wanted to say "NO, I DID NOT DO A BREAK AND ENTRY AND STEAL FILES!" but I restrained myself.

Just when I thought it couldn't get any worse, I took another body blow. When I became sick, I had to face many losses, but the loss of a couple of our closest friends was not one I could have ever anticipated. When Bill and I met Tim and Nancy we instantly connected and became the best of friends. We did all the things good friends enjoy like playing cards, laughing around the campfire, walks and vacationing together. I thought this friendship would last a lifetime. However, as a quote I once read says, "Some people come in your life as blessings, others come in your life as lessons." There were definitely lessons to be learned from this friendship. As I reflect back on what was, it saddens me that it didn't last. I've come to realize it was a friendship that wasn't meant to be one for a lifetime.

I had noticed that Nancy was treating me differently. She was distant when we were together, and I sensed that something wasn't right. In hindsight, I should have addressed my concerns with her but, as I was very stressed, I just didn't have the energy to add more pressure on myself so I tried to ignore the situation.

I had been off work for a few weeks and was extremely sick. On an afternoon when I was feeling quite ill, the phone rang. I was shocked to hear Tim say, "Debbie, you owe Nancy an apology. You hurt her and she's really upset." I couldn't comprehend what he was taking about. I became hysterical. I began to realize it was because Nancy had asked me to disclose something related to a couple we both knew, but I had given my word to keep what I knew confidential. It was an immediate trigger for me and was the end of the friendship.

I now understand that hearing Tim make a false accusation was a trigger for me. It was not Tim that I heard; it was Jim. I regressed back to my childhood, back to the defenseless little girl who was being accused of something she didn't do. I felt helpless. I was distraught. I've taken away many lessons from that experience, the most important of which is to not allow myself to be put in the middle of other people's problems.

When it felt like everything was crashing around me, something positive came out of nowhere. I'm a believer that people come into our lives for a reason and at the time they are meant to. I was desperate to feel better and willing to try almost anything. I saw an ad for one-hour evening sessions with Damian Dyke entitled "Trauma/Tension Relief Exercises" (TRE®). The "Trauma" part of it spoke to me immediately. I knew I couldn't participate in a group session so I took a chance and contacted Damian to see if he would do private sessions with me. Not only did he agree to private sessions in my home but he brought his own blue gym mat for me. I didn't know what to expect, but my gut said I could trust him.

Damian explained that he was not a certified TRE® practitioner, but when he was in the military he suffered from back pain and a friend introduced him to TRE®. After a number of sessions he had relief from his pain and wanted to share his newfound knowledge with others. Damian's group sessions attracted people who were interested in relieving stress and tension, which TRE® does. I was still "in the closet" about my mental illness but something told me to put my trust in Damian, and I did. I explained some of my history on the phone and a little more when he came to my home. I felt comfortable and was not judged.

Damian showed me how to do warm up exercises prior to his introduction of TRE®, on his blue gym mat. He explained they would help my body release stress, tension and trauma which had built up over time. He instructed me to lay on my back, bend my knees and lift my pelvis. As I held this position I felt trembling begin in my face that moved to my arms and legs. In no time my whole body was shaking, and I began to cry inexplicably. Damian, a natural instructor, took it all in stride. He was patient, understanding and compassionate. I instinctively knew he had been sent to me for a purpose. It only took a few sessions with Damian's coaching before I felt ready to practice TRE® on my own.

I practiced TRE® every couple of days for a few months, and it helped let go of chronic tension in my body. Then, as with many things we learn, the novelty wore off. Although I wasn't ready to commit to a regular practice of TRE®, I knew it was another tool I could turn to for healing when I was ready.

I continued to receive Short Term Disability Insurance through my employer. Insurance representatives were in constant contact with me. I was fortunate to have an understanding and compassionate case manager, and I knew all too well that if I didn't have all my i's dotted and t's crossed, my insurance could be cut off. It was often my role at work to advocate for employees who were denied insurance, so I was comfortable with the insurance process—until I received notification from Manulife that a psychiatrist from Moncton would be visiting Labrador City. I was required to attend an appointment with her for an Independent Medical Examination (IME).

In all my years working with this employer, side by side with the Human Resources and Occupational Health Departments, a psychiatrist was never brought to Labrador City to complete an IME for an employee with a mental illness. Was I being paranoid? Maybe. Was I reading between the lines, seeing that someone in authority believed I was "faking it"? Yes. Can I prove it? No. Have I learned to listen to my gut? Yes. Need I say anything further?

I was distraught; the stress of knowing I was being scrutinized by my employer made my mental health deteriorate. How could a company I had given so much of myself to treat me this way? I needed validation, not mistrust. I felt humiliated as I walked into my appointment at The Two Seasons Inn. It was the first time I'd seen a psychiatrist, and I knew it would be difficult. Under these conditions, however, it was more exhausting than I could ever have imagined.

In order to do her assessment, Dr. Barbara Ross had to ask difficult questions, ones which required me to relive some of my trauma. Until I had to leave work in February, I was able to push the effects of my trauma down. As the bricks that weighed my feelings down began to crumble, there came a point where I could no longer hold them in place. I initially felt threatened by the psychiatrist before I even met her, but she alleviated any misgivings I had. She showed me understanding, caring, concern and, most importantly, respect. I left with my dignity intact at the end of our three-hour assessment. If my employer was "out to get me," they hired the wrong psychiatrist. Dr. Ross was the first person to validate what I had suspected all along but didn't want to admit. She diagnosed me with Complex Post Traumatic Stress Disorder (C-PTSD).

Many professionals are educated about PTSD but not C-PTSD. The "Complex" aspect is important as it distinguishes this mental illness from PTSD, which occurs from a single traumatizing event. C-PTSD occurs most often in individuals who have been severely abused or neglected in childhood. The severe trauma interrupts psychologic and neurologic development in the child. When an adult is traumatized they usually have the tools to deal with the trauma.

My family doctor arranged for me to see Dr. Walsh, a psychiatrist who visited Labrador on a regular basis. It required me to make two trips to Happy Valley-Goose Bay where Dr. Walsh conducted an assessment and confirmed Dr. Ross' diagnosis. Although C-PTSD is a fairly new concept and not fully understood by mental health professionals, I saw a glimpse of light at the end of the tunnel. Dr. Walsh gave me hope in knowing that I may finally get some relief from the unrelenting agony I was experiencing.

Politics is something that has always been of interest to me, and I was elected to Labrador City's town council in 2009. When I put my name on the ballot for town council I thought it could be a good starting point, as I had hoped to pursue some sort of involvement in this area when I retired. After becoming ill, I pushed myself to attend council meetings, but sitting through a meeting became more and more difficult, and I was overwhelmed with the intensity of concentration that was required to conduct the business of the town. The exhaustion was crippling; the amount of energy it took to pretend I was "normal" was unbearable.

I am not a quitter. When I take on something I persevere until the task is finished. I wanted to finish my four-year term on town council, but I had to face reality; I was just too sick. I sat at my computer to write my letter of resignation, tears streaming down my cheeks. My life as I had pictured it was slowly fading before my eyes, and I was helpless to change it.

As difficult as it was, I knew I had to accept that I was too sick to work and major changes were in store. The time had come to apply for Long Term Disability (LTD) and Canada Pension Plan Disability (CPP). Through all the "fog," tears and confusion, I completed the applications. Thankfully, both my LTD and CPP were approved immediately.

Major Life Changes

Then another storm hit without warning. William was just getting his life back together when Wabush Mines, his employer for almost nine years, shut their doors for good. The Wabush Mines closure greatly affected our family because Bram also lost his livelihood, and it was a major loss for all of Labrador West. Nearly four hundred people were out of work, which also affected dozens of businesses that were dependent on the mine.

Bill and I decided to downsize, sold our townhouse and bought a mini home that was to be our retirement home in Labrador City. Our family has always been very close, and we wanted to be where our children were, but the mine closure paired with my mental illness changed our plans. We had recently decided to close our family business and sell a couple of rental properties so it was time to make a major life change.

We sold our mini home, packed up our belongings and left our home of nearly forty years. It was a difficult decision, but Bill and I knew that if I didn't leave Labrador I would never be able to start the healing process. There were too many triggers there which interfered with my well-being. My friend, Line, had said to Bill, "You have to get Debbie out of there or she'll never get better." She was right; I could not heal in a triggering environment.

As we packed our possessions, it was also a time to purge. We sold, gave away or trashed many personal things, but when I looked at the blue gym mat Damian had given me I hesitated to toss it. Something was telling me to keep it, so I did. I had no idea the significance of the blue gym mat but I would find out.

Bill's sisters live on the east coast of Newfoundland, so we considered building a home there to be close to family. Deep down I knew I couldn't live on the east coast and be near the place where so much trauma had occurred. To this day, I cannot return to my childhood home in Burnside because it stirs up too much pain which, in turn, causes anxiety, flashbacks and seizures. Prior to my illness, Bill and I had many discussions about where and when we would retire. These discussions always ended the same because we couldn't decide where we would go.

Line married Melv Gale whose hometown is Hampden, NL. When they retired and left Labrador, they moved to a little community of five families, just outside the town of Hampden, on a small road called Fox Point. All five houses are on one side of the road. During a game of cards on one of their visits to Labrador City, Line told us about a beautiful piece of property across the road from their house. She had walked up through the thick trees on the hill and discovered a flat area of land at the top that overlooked the ocean.

"Deb, if I could take our house and move it up there, I would," she said. "It is breathtaking."

The moment Line finished her sentence, I jumped up from the table and called the Crown Lands office in Corner Brook. I instinctively knew that piece of land was going to be ours. Our friends found this quite funny because I had mercilessly teased them about living in the "boonies" when they moved to Fox Point. In all seriousness, I never pictured myself living in the "boonies." Interestingly, anyone could have bought the piece of land in question, but it was uninhabited. It was the most amazing place, with an astonishing view of the ocean. I believe that fate brought this healing place to me; it was just meant to be.

During the following year I communicated back and forth with Dean Abbott of Adventure Log Homes until we had finalized plans for our dream home on Fox Point. We moved from Labrador City in May 2014. Our home for the next five months would be in our travel trailer that was parked in Line and Melv's driveway across from our soon-to-be home.

William, now unemployed, decided to move to Fox Point with us. His relationship with Lynn had ended, so there was nothing to keep him in Labrador City. With his newfound sobriety, hanging out with his sober dad was good for William. He was a great help for us, as he was Bill's right-hand man. Together they put in a driveway, cleared the land, put in a water and sewer system, built a garage and created a family/guest apartment in the basement. I had no idea what was involved in building a new home; it was quite the undertaking.

Adventure Log Homes did not disappoint. They were responsible for construction of the home, and we were required to complete the excavation, foundation, electrical and plumbing. I co-ordinated the construction of our home but, with the condition of my mental health, it was very challenging. However, the people we hired for the various jobs were second to none. We sure lucked out with every aspect of the construction of our new home.

On October 10, 2014, we moved into our log home on Fox Point. It is the only home on one side of the road upon a huge hill overlooking White Bay. It has a million-dollar view and is my healing place. The quiet beauty of nature surrounding us has helped bring me to a place of peacefulness that I never dreamed possible. It's a little piece of heaven right here on Earth.

After we moved from Labrador to Newfoundland I made every effort to find appropriate help in the Deer Lake/Corner Brook area, without success. A couple of experiences with counsellors and a psychiatrist set me back in my healing, as they had no understanding of how to treat my illness. Thankfully, as a counsellor I recognized the damage that was being done. My heart aches for people with this illness who are unable to receive proper help. I've always been a mental health advocate. Firstly, it was in my career as a counsellor. I never expected that I would have to advocate for proper services for my own mental health. When I couldn't get suitable assistance from staff at Western Health, I took my concerns up the ladder, without success.

I felt it was important that the public understand the lack of appropriate mental health services with Western Health, so I spoke to CBC about my concerns. The story was aired on CBC's *Here and Now* program as well as on CBC's website. I had talked to Ruby prior to doing the interview, and she knew the concerns I had with Western Health. I had not planned how the interview would proceed, but I just went with the flow, responding to the questions the reporter asked in an open and honest way. I wasn't aware of the spin she would put on the story or the headline that would be used.

The reporter said, "Her PTSD was caused by a traumatic childhood and gang-related activity from when she lived in Ontario." She used my statement, "I felt very abandoned. When you have trauma in your childhood, abandonment is an issue." I have done numerous public stories, including interviews for TV with CBC, and had always told Ruby about these interviews. I expected to hear from her once she saw the story and thought it strange that I hadn't received a call until a few days after it aired. Her words are forever etched in my mind: "I heard your interview. I don't like it. Everyone here knows me. I'm embarrassed. If I treated you that bad, don't ever speak to me again!" CLICK! I held the phone in my hand and looked at it in disbelief; I was shocked.

I sent Ruby a message saying that the interview was not about her, that it was about the lack of care provided by Western Health which made me feel abandoned. When I was a child I was abandoned by my parents. It's a feeling that I've carried with me and shows up unexpectedly in other situations, especially when you add in a mental illness. In the interview I didn't say that Ruby treated me badly. It's unfortunate that she couldn't understand where I was coming from. She saw the story from her perspective, and that's something I can't change. That was six years ago, and I have not heard from or seen her since.

I can't understand what upset her so much. She knew I had talked publicly about my childhood, as I had told her about the occasions I had shared my story. The difference this time was that she heard for herself what I had said so many times before. I can only assume this was the reason she decided to disown me. Searching for an understanding of why this woman abandoned me has left me bewildered; whatever her reason, it's beyond my comprehension.

I was deeply saddened that I had lost Ruby again. At first I was in shock and disbelief, and I realized I was grieving the loss of Ruby. As the stages of grief kicked in I began to bargain. I wrote the following message to her:

Mom, I want you to know that I miss talking to you. I also want you to know that I really appreciate the things we have shared which are so special to me, like being able to sit here and crochet because you taught me how; like being able to sew and mend clothes (even though I don't like doing it); like remembering you every time I make a boiled raisin cake because you liked to sit and lick off the spoon; like being able to talk to you about things other girls couldn't talk to their moms about; like being able to talk to you about my sister because you're the only one who understands. Thank you for the good times and the love you have shown me.

It's taken me a long time to grieve losing Ruby. I've heard some say it's easier to grieve when the person you've lost is dead. This makes sense to me as it's still difficult to know that she is only a few hours away from me and I can't see her. I've ridden a roller coaster of emotions. She has made the choice to cut me out of her life, and I can only assume she is better off without me. I'm sure I caused her stress, but I hope she has found peace.

To add insult to injury, after receiving Ruby's phone call, I then received the following message from David:

> "well i seen your interview its not very nice making mom out to be a bad person i think yourshould look at at your familey a drunk for a son and a daughter the looks shes anorexia i have to daughters that spend more time with mom an do more for mom than your kids ever did an will do they both got good jobs then theres bernie she looks out to mom not like you you dont evencome to see her for what reasons i dont no well then if something ever happen to mom you probley never ever no untill its to late i could say more"

This was my response to David before he blocked me:
You have no idea what you're talking about. You did not live the life I did. So, go ahead. Say more. Dig the knife a little deeper.

The "Bernie and daughters" David references in his message are his second wife and her daughters. I attempted to be friends with her, but I always felt I just wasn't her cup of tea. We've had some disagreements over the years, and any attempt at a relationship ended when she wrote me a message in which she made false accusations about me and fired unnecessary insults which cut deep. In her message, for example, she references an annual Christmas letter which I sent to family and friends as "nothing more than a brag letter." That hurt to the point that I've never again written an annual Christmas letter. She made it clear she wants nothing to do with me.

This was the third time my family has abandoned me, and I imagine it will be the last. The first came when they gave me to CAS in Ontario, the second after Jim was killed in the car accident. Ruby is in her 80s, and it has been six years since her phone call that ended our relationship. David and Bernie hate the ground I walk on. Jim is dead. So, there it is, a family gone!

Each year as Mother's Day approaches, I feel a sadness, a dread, an emptiness, an ache, and occasionally anger surfaces. In years gone by I forced myself to pick out an "appropriate" Mother's Day card that basically said nothing. I felt guilty that I couldn't send her a card that showered her with love, gratitude and honour. Since being disowned, for the third and final time, I avoid the aisle full of Mother's Day cards. As I heal from severe traumas, I am working toward forgiveness. It's not an acceptance for what was or what was not done by my mother but a letting go of what has caused me anguish. I sincerely hope that her son, daughter-in-law and step-grandchildren give her memorable Mother's Days. She has been a mother and grandmother to them, as she could not be to me, nor my children.

The outpouring of love I receive from my own children every day, not just Mother's Day, more than compensates for the loss of my biological mother. With their ongoing support and understanding I realize how truly blessed I am.

An Addition to the Family

William moved into our family/guest basement apartment when we built our home on Fox Point. He worked a few jobs but was on the lookout for something better and eventually found employment with Muskrat Falls in Labrador. Before William flew to Muskrat Falls he spent a few days in Labrador City with Lynn and they got back together.

Next came one of the most heartwarming announcements that has ever filled my ears: Lynn and William were having a baby! Because Lisa and Bram had been unsuccessful and William had stated that he never wanted to have a child, I had given up hope of ever becoming a grandmother.

One of the happiest days of my life was December 18, 2016, the birth of our precious grandson, William Lawrence Samson. He is named William to carry on the "Bill Samson" tradition which originated from Flat Island, Bill's birthplace. There was never a doubt in William's mind that his son would be named after him.

I will forever remember nervously sitting in the waiting area outside the delivery room at the hospital in Labrador City. Having Line and Melv with us made the waiting more bearable, as we had many laughs, which is always the case when we're together. The moment William emerged from the delivery room with his son swaddled in his arms, my eyes welled up with tears of joy. Seeing the pride and delight shine in William's eyes brought more exhilaration than I could have imagined. There was a glow on his face like I had never seen before. An intense love, different than any I could have imagined, flowed over me.

Our new grandson was the best Christmas present we've ever received. I had crocheted a Santa hat and cocoon for his first Christmas picture. He looked so perfect in it, and I showered my Facebook page with pictures.

On Christmas Eve, William Lawrence was dedicated into the Christian faith. He wore his great grandfather's christening dress which has been passed down through the generations. As I held him in my arms, I felt the loving presence of Mr. Samson (Bill's father). I know he would have wanted to have another Samson wearing the family heirloom. Mr. Samson's parents bought him the christening dress in 1916, the year he was born and christened, and here we were one hundred years later. It was a magical occasion, in a packed church, with both families present to witness our precious baby boy being welcomed into God's family.

William had moved back to Labrador City with Lynn, which was a dilemma for Bill and me. When we decided to leave Labrador City and move to Fox Point we had no intention of returning. Now we had a new grandson and both him and our son were in Labrador City. William suggested we move back to Labrador City, but this just wasn't an option as we had settled into our new home on Fox Point.

"Your grandson will never know you," he said.

"I can assure you that he will know who I am, and I will be a presence in his life," I responded.

Remembering how important and special my grandmother was to me has made me determined to always be a part of William Lawrence's (we call him William Lawrence to distinguish the difference between him and his dad) life, and I've kept my word. I fly or drive to Labrador City at least four or five times a year, and we FaceTime almost daily. William Lawrence knows who Nana and Poppy Samson are and how much he is loved.

When I spend time with my grandson I have to be careful not to get overstimulated, which could result in a seizure. I also have to be careful and have a plan in place in the event that I am triggered. He's an active little guy, but I'm well enough to care for him for a few hours before I need to rest.

On one occasion while playing with William Lawrence, he unexpectedly began calling me "Nannie" while we were home alone.

"Nannie, Nannie, Nannie, Nannie..." he sang.

Even before he was born I made it known that I wanted to be called Nana, not Nannie, without realizing that hearing "Nannie" would be a trigger for me. I felt a rush of emotions intensifying so quickly I thought I couldn't control them. Flashbacks of happy moments with my grandmother played in front of me like I was watching a movie. She was my world; I miss her so much. I fought back tears until Bill came home, then I let it all flow uncontrollably. I'm grateful for this moment, as difficult as it was, but that's how triggers are; they make you face them. Facing my triggers has been healing. If William Lawrence calls me Nannie again, it won't be as painful.

William Lawrence is four years old now, a magical age. I get to be a kid again when I'm with him. He's such a smart, funny, strong-willed and loving little guy. I thoroughly enjoy the fun we have together.

While playing with him in his bedroom he wanted us, his toys and my little dog to pretend we were sleeping in his bed. He turned off the lights, and we made snoring noises. Then he made an alarm clock sound, said it was time to get up, jumped out of bed and turned on the light. He looked at me and said, "Nana, did you shit yourself?" I couldn't move in the bed, as I laughed so hard that my stomach hurt. He's my pride and joy, and I have a love for him that is like no other.

William is now a single dad. When I reflect on where he's come from, through addiction and challenges in his life, I'm filled with pride to see the remarkable father he has become. Recovery from addiction is one of the most difficult things William has ever done. He worked hard to get where he is although it wasn't always easy. William Lawrence will, one day, realize just what an amazing dad he has; one who can conquer anything life throws at him.

Complex Post-Traumatic Stress Disorder Effects

When I was put off work in February 2012, I became sicker with each day, especially as the developments of the EFAP office closure unfolded. I've often said my employer sent me over the edge because the events that preceded the closure of the EFAP office triggered C-PTSD symptoms that were buried and manageable and caused them to worsen. I wanted to believe that I would get well, that I would soon return to active employment. Fate, however, had dealt me a different hand.

I saw a counsellor from the local mental health department. I was unable to go to the hospital as I was too ill, so she came to my home. My first counsellor, Annette Parsons, is a dear friend. She knew me well and was able to provide the support and guidance I needed at a time when I was barely able to function. I was devastated when Annette told me she was moving. It's challenging to move from one counsellor to another, especially because I lived in a small town where everyone knew me. The bad experiences I've had with other counsellors made me skeptical to let another one into my life. I knew, however, that I needed help and could not heal on my own.

I decided to put aside any doubts and fears I had and give someone else a chance to help me. As I reflect on my apprehension I now realize that another person was put into my life at exactly the right time and place. My new counsellor, who wishes to remain anonymous as she is too modest, has been with me since December 2012. She is an expert in the treatment of C-PTSD. I don't know where I'd be without her; she knows me intimately and has helped me beyond expectation.

Complex PTSD is difficult to treat, and the counsellor has to be specifically trained in this area. I've heard that soldiers get PTSD from war, and children grow up and get C-PTSD from the war at home, which means that violent homes have the same effect on children's brains as combat on soldiers. Lilly Hope Lucario gives one of the best definitions of C-PTSD: "A severe psychiatric disorder caused by ongoing, or repeated interpersonal trauma (abuse), suffered within a captivity environment where the victim perceives no means of escape. It requires highly specialized trauma informed empathic treatment, to address all the pervasive complex symptoms." Jim said he had "straightened me out" after he abandoned me to the "care" of CAS. No, Jim, YOU DID NOT STRAIGHTEN ME OUT, YOU FUCKED ME UP!!!

Prior to C-PTSD I felt great satisfaction in being able to organize and remember things that needed to get done. People could count on me to ensure plans were made and followed through on, so it upset me when I realized my memory was no longer functioning as it once did. I remember, with sadness, the first time it hit me that my memory was affected by my mental illness. In our group of friends I was usually the one who would organize trips, dinners, etc., and I prided myself on being dependable. One time, however, I mixed up the details of the trip. When Bill and I went to meet up with Line and Melv they weren't where I thought they were going to be. I was puzzled. Upon making contact with them, Line said, "Deb, that's not where you told us to meet." I was confused and could have sworn she was mixed up. When the others told me I was the one who had it mixed up, I began to realize that it was, indeed, my mistake.

I'm not saying I've never made a mistake; I have made many. This was different though. I had planned and organized a trip for these same friends to Las Vegas, including all the shows, hotels, flights, etc. How could I mix up a simple trip to Gros Morne? Things that were once routine and came automatically to me were no longer. I couldn't remember when to take my medication, and I forgot simple tasks such as feeding my service dog. As time went on, my memory worsened to the point that in order to get things accomplished I had to depend on others to remind me. My house was plastered with sticky notes reminding me what I was supposed to be doing. Sometimes I even forgot to read the sticky notes.

Lately, I have noticed some improvement in my memory. I no longer need sticky notes as reminders to take my medication on time. I still like to organize and make plans, but I do it differently now. I ensure it is written down, and I have become accustomed to rechecking and double checking. Essentially, I have learned a new way of being; it could be much worse. I think of the people who have dementia and remind myself I am blessed. I just have to be more patient with myself. I truly believe I'm on the road to healing the hippocampus in my brain, which is responsible for memory.

Growing up in a home with violence that no child should ever witness caused permanent changes to my young, developing brain. My body was stuck in stress response. Living in a relentless state of threat naturally causes one's body to go into survival mode, which fractures the mind and takes away the person's peace. It leaves the mind and body stuck in horror. This chronic stress has had long-term effects on my health. It is exhausting when we are wired to constantly look for threats, be hypervigilant and expect the worst because the worst is all we've known. The hormones which flood through our bodies from the arousal of our sympathetic nervous system help us scan for threats but also make us tired. One cannot live in a constant state of arousal without long-term side effects.

As I got older I developed the ability to stuff my stress and feelings down. It was natural for me and was all I knew. It was how I survived.

As I grew into an adult, I noticed things about myself that were "different." I was unable to tolerate certain sounds, for example. I had no idea this could be related to C-PTSD. Snoring gave me extreme anxiety to the point I had to give up sleeping with Bill, an extremely loud snorer. I was so embarrassed because I thought it was shameful to sleep separately from my husband. I didn't talk about it, and I was concerned I would be judged for not loving him if I couldn't sleep with him. I've since learned that hypersensitivity to certain sounds is a characteristic of C-PTSD. Now we talk openly about it and even laugh that I "tuck Bill in" when he goes to bed. Generally, I've been able to find ways of coping with the sound of snoring. I sleep with a white noise machine, which drowns out Bill's snoring in a next-door room.

My biggest issue is with Reggie, my daughter's English Bulldog. He snores excessively. I feel my body becoming tense when he snores. My thinking becomes confused, my eyelids start to flutter and I start to tremble. I know a full-blown seizure is on the way if I can't escape Reggie's piercing noise. I am blessed to have the most understanding daughter and son-in-law. It breaks my heart that there is always an issue for me with

Reggie's snoring, and I was scared they wouldn't want me to visit them or they would stop visiting me. Some would; but not Lisa and Bram. They turn Reggie on his side, play with him, pet him, prop up his head—anything they can think of to help. I am so appreciative of the empathy they show toward me and my mental illness.

I have had severe insomnia for years. I would lie on the couch in the living room watching TV until I drifted off most nights. I tried all of the known treatments: go to bed at the same time, wake up at the same time, don't nap, avoid caffeine, etc. Nothing worked. Bill saw this wearing me down so he suggested I ask my doctor for something to help. I didn't want to take pills because I didn't want to become dependent on them.

"Deb," Bill finally said, "you're fifty years old. So what if you become dependent? So what if you have to take them for the rest of your life?"

This, coming from an alcoholic who fully understands what it's like to be dependent, made me think. It was the beginning of the end of insomnia. Yes, I can't sleep without pills. Do I feel better? Yes. Do I wish I had done it a long time ago? Yes. Better late than never.

I thought I had escaped vicarious trauma until one day when my son and I were having a conversation about a friend who is a front-line worker and is required to have regular Critical Incident Stress Debriefings as a means of preventing PTSD or vicarious trauma. My mind suddenly flashed back to the first time I had to deal with the suicide of an employee.

I relived the phone call I received from the police as I was leaving my home to go to work. The officer informed me of the suicide. He then advised me that the mother of the employee was asking for me to visit her at home. Not only was the young man who died an employee, he was also a friend of our family. I was devastated. I fought to hold back the tears and forced myself to hold it together during the home visit.

As I walked to my car, a friend was walking toward me. He had just heard of the suicide.

"I don't know how I'm going to get through this," I said to him.

He said, "Just say a prayer and God will walk with you."

I did as he suggested and there was definitely a power greater than myself guiding me through the days ahead, as I found a strength I didn't realize I had.

Five years ago the mother whom I visited wrote on my Facebook timeline:

Hi Debbie. You are a very special friend. You have helped us in our hard times and I will never forget it. You are a very special person. Take care. Love you so much.

As I've done with the other traumatic episodes in my life, I stuffed this one down and tried not to feel. This was the first of countless overwhelming and traumatic events I dealt with during my career as a counsellor. I try not to think about them, but there are occasions when something will trigger a memory. I have the stories of hundreds of people stored in my mind, and they have become a part of me. One cannot listen to upwards of twenty-five years of other's stories without some impact on their well-being.

It took many, many years for me to learn to sleep in the dark. Being in a dark room was a major trigger for me because much of my sexual abuse took place in the dark, so I assume that's the connection. I was terrified if I awoke in the dark. I needed to have a small light on. I remember being at university without a nightlight and no bedside light in the room. I slept with the large florescent light on until I got to a store. It was too bright, but it was better than experiencing the terror of awaking in the dark.

Not only was I fearful of sleeping in the dark, but I was also afraid to actually go to sleep; it's a real thing called somniphobia. "Oh, the terrible struggle that I have had against sleep so often of late," says author Brian Stoker. "The pain of the sleeplessness, or the pain of the fear of sleep, and with such unknown horror as it has for me! How blessed are some people, whose lives have no fears, no dreads; to whom sleep is a blessing that comes nightly, and brings nothing but sweet dreams." I look forward to the day when I actually "want" to go to sleep. My husband is always so happy when it's bedtime; I want that. I'm fearful because my body and subconscious remember the nights of trauma and the nightmares. Putting my head on a pillow and sleeping means losing control.

A couple of years ago, an inexplicable miracle occurred. Most nights I can now put my head on the pillow with no fear, anxiety or panic attacks. Occasionally that little fear creeps in, but it doesn't last long. I still procrastinate at bedtime because it's almost as if I'm expecting "it" to happen, but my somniphobia is not as common as it once was.

Since I've been unable to work, my sleeping routine has changed significantly. I sleep from 3 a.m. to 11 a.m., and I like this schedule as I function better in the night; I've never been a morning person. The new sleeping routine evolved because I wanted to avoid going to sleep. I was very tense and nervous, even wishing I could survive without sleep. I was trying to escape the terrifying C-PTSD nightmares that shake me to the core. My past traumas revisited me in my sleep, waking me in the middle of a panic attack, giving me flashbacks and unpleasant body sensations. These night terrors were relentless and were at their worst prior to my diagnosis of C-PTSD and for a short while after the diagnosis. They have subsided since I've been receiving treatment.

When I went for sexual abuse counselling I heard the other survivors in my group talk about flashbacks. I understood the concept but was thankful I had not experienced them. After listening to their descriptions, I hoped I never would. A couple of years after being diagnosed with C-PTSD, to my horror I began having flashbacks and reliving the horrendous experiences of my trauma. There is a large picture of a wolf on the wall of our living room, and when the flashbacks occurred, I was looking at the picture as if it were a movie screen. Visions of my trauma replayed before my eyes, and I was helpless to stop them. My body experienced a repeat performance of the stress response: the fear and terror, the feeling of being trapped, the physical sensations and intense emotions. It was an out-of-body experience from which I couldn't escape. I wanted to run but I was frozen in time.

Chronic anxiety that often appears out of the blue is one of the major symptoms I experience because of C-PTSD. It's like an invasion of my body and brain. A tsunami of debilitating sensations rush over me from the tip of my toes to the top of my head. I become confused and feel trembling under my skin. I try to push it away, but I rarely can without an Ativan or Clonazepam.

Depression and mood swings go hand in hand with C-PTSD as well. In the early stages of my diagnosis, I was in a deep, dark place and being dragged further and further down. I was helpless and could not pull myself back out. I was trapped; I was not me anymore. I was exhausted to the point that sleep couldn't fix it. I felt a paralyzing numbness and craved comfort from my family and friends, but it was a double-edged sword. I needed people but I no longer had the ability to socialize, and pushing myself only made me sicker. I was once the person who attended public functions and got involved in community events, but at that point I was unable to drag myself out of the house. I was a prisoner in my own body.

Avoidance is a significant behaviour in people with C-PTSD. It took me some time to realize I unconsciously used avoidance to escape the memories and feelings associated with being in certain places and situations. In that nasty message I received from David he said, in part, "You don't even come to see her, for what reasons I don't know. Well then, if something ever happens to Mom you will never even know, until it's too late." I was angry with him for his cruel words, but as I've had time to reflect on the part regarding not visiting Ruby, he is absolutely right. Prior to her disowning me, I avoided visiting her, particularly after I was diagnosed with C-PTSD and my illness became increasingly worse. Ruby lives in Gander. I experienced severe anxiety when Bill and I drove past Gander on the Trans-Canada Highway. As my illness progressed and I began having seizures, it was the thought of David, Ruby, Gander, Burnside and Jim which would trigger a seizure, so I began avoiding anything connected to the abuse I suffered as a child. It was impossible to avoid everything, but the things I could control, however, I did avoid.

If only there was a way to know what will trigger me. I'm learning some triggers, but I'll never live long enough to learn and avoid all of them. One time I was using an electric chopper to chop onions when it suddenly stopped. I thought I had put too much onion in it and broke it, but when Bill inspected it (he is a great Mr. Fix-It) he discovered it had tripped the circuit. Although Bill assured me I hadn't broken the chopper, my brain interpreted the event differently, and I began having a seizure. I later recognized it was because my body remembered how Jim would react when I did something wrong—the yelling, swearing, belittling, threatening and criticism would have flooded my mind and triggered fight/flight/freeze.

Even as I write about the chopper incident I feel a sense of "dread" sweep over my entire body, and I wonder if it will ever go away. I'm determined to never give up. I'll face them, one trigger at a time, and get through this. I will not let my abusers win. I will face each trigger as it comes, and I will no longer use avoidance to cope. I've learned that I must face my triggers, as difficult as it is, in order to heal.

As my C-PTSD progressed, my ability to concentrate became severely reduced. I was no longer able to watch TV or read. Even the simplest of conversations became increasingly more difficult. My lack of concentration began long before I was diagnosed with C-PTSD and became so serious that I was incapable of performing at work. I had to depend on my co-worker, Pam, to assist me with presentations and workshops. After about half an hour, I would think to myself, *Here comes the fog*. It was devastating to realize that something was happening to me, and I fought to hide my confusion, but I sensed it becoming worse. I was scared as it became more and more difficult to hide my cognitive impairment. I didn't know what was happening to my brain. At the end of a work day I went home and cried from exhaustion.

Before the onset of my mental illness, I was passionate about continuous learning. I took courses, new programs or workshops in an effort to expand my knowledge. I honestly believed I would be a life-long learner, but when my ability to concentrate evaporated I was forced to stop learning. Suddenly, who I was and who I wanted to become was taken from me. Accepting this fate was challenging. I'm still grieving the loss of who I was, but I'm learning to accept a new version of me. She's not who I had anticipated, but I like her.

I began having panic attacks long before I was educated about them. I now realize that I had been having them most of my adult life. I called them my "I gotta get out of here feeling." I was embarrassed about these incidents and learned to mask them when they came unexpectedly if I felt trapped, if there was no window in the room or I couldn't see a door, if I was in a dark room, if the area was too small or crowded, or if a person was talking too much and I was forced to listen. The list goes on. My place of employment was an enormous challenge. I was required to be in many situations which brought on panic attacks. My boss's office had no windows, and I often wonder how I managed to be in such a state and hide it; it was exhausting and increasingly difficult. I became a great actress but, to this day, I don't know how I managed to do it.

In May 2005, I had the good fortune of attending the Canadian Traumatic Stress Network National Forum in Ottawa. I decided to take in a two-day pre-forum workshop entitled "The Psychobiology of Trauma: A New Paradigm for Working with Trauma" that was presented by Jeannette Ambrose. This was my introduction to Self Regulation Therapy (SRT)—a whole new field of interest for me. Ms. Ambrose's words spoke to me. At one point she asked for a volunteer so she could demonstrate SRT; I was eager to help and happily raised my hand.

For many years I couldn't get the fog to lift from my head, at least not permanently. It was especially heavy and affected my cognitive abilities when I flew. Although I had an extreme fear of flying which left me trembling under constant panic attacks, I refused to let the fear win. So here I was at a forum in Ottawa in an intense fog on display for an audience while a therapist showed how SRT is practiced. Jeanette asked me to sense into the activation in my body. When I closed my eyes and tracked the sensations in my body I noticed tingling and heat. She asked me to track how it felt and moved, and to just allow it to do what it needed to do. This short activity allowed me to discharge a very small amount of incomplete fight/flight/freeze response that had built up in my nervous system. Just this small release brought relief. After taking my seat I felt the fog gradually diminish; I experienced an energy that I had forgotten even existed. I was sold on SRT!

After the presentation I stayed behind to learn more about this intriguing therapy for myself and my clients at work. I asked Jeannette if she would spend more time with me after the workshop and she generously agreed. I wasn't sure what to expect from the SRT sessions but I was eager to find out. To my delight, I was not required to talk about my trauma. She asked me a few questions, although I don't remember what they were. She then led me to focus on sensations in my body. I recall trembling, tingling and, eventually, all out shaking; there were tears and then laughter. I felt safe as Jeannette guided me through the process of observing my body sensations. After our time together I was relaxed and in a peaceful place in my mind.

Prior to SRT with Jennette, I experienced an overall body pain from the tips of my toes to the top of my head. This pain intensified when I had to be on my feet. Cooking a meal, for example, was unbearable. A rheumatologist diagnosed "fibromyalgia-like symptoms." After therapy with Jennette this pain disappeared. She helped me release tension in my muscles. Years of trauma caused my nervous system to be in a constant state of reactivity, so I was unable to relax and the fight/flight stress response was constantly engaged. After this remarkable experience with SRT, I was determined to learn more. I had an exceptionally supportive boss at the time, and she didn't hesitate to grant me permission to be trained as a Self Regulation Therapist.

The closest training was being held in Winnipeg, which meant travelling back and forth over a two-year period. The intense training also included personal therapy. Winnipeg, training, therapy and travel were things I looked forward to. I booked private therapy sessions with Dr. Edward Josephs and Dr. Lynne Zettl, the trainers/psychologists and developers of SRT, each time I went to Winnipeg. These two individuals became near and dear to my heart. Through their therapy I was able to discharge a lot of the activation in my nervous system that was caused by the enormous amount of trauma in my life. Through SRT I overcame my fear of flying, but the big bonus was no more panic attacks! I am forever grateful to Ed and Lynne for their help.

I brought my new skills back to work and helped many employees. I was, and to the best of my knowledge, still am, the only Self Regulation Therapist east of Manitoba. The education Dr. Josephs and Dr. Zettl provided through the Canadian Foundation for Trauma Research & Education (CFTRE) was profound. It not only enabled me to help others, but it also helped me to better understand myself. Unfortunately for me, these two brilliant psychologists live on the other side of Canada, in British Columbia.

Psychogenic Non-Epileptic Seizures (PNES)

My psychiatrist prescribed a variety of medications for me in an effort to treat the C-PTSD. I'm overly cautious when I try a new one because of the horrendous side effects some of them have caused.

In March of 2016 I started taking Risperidone. With each passing day I became more and more confused and my memory worsened. I felt as if my brain was in "fast forward" and I couldn't slow my thoughts. I talked continuously, excitedly and uncontrollably. While hiking with Line on a beautiful, sunny afternoon, we met a couple of men we knew on snowmobiles. There was a badge on one man's coat that said Wade, but his name isn't Wade (he was wearing his brother's coat). I made a big deal over it, used words that were uncustomary and laughed uncontrollably. I came up with ideas which were not normal for me, although they seemed natural at the time. The situation didn't warrant my unusual reaction, and I feel a sense of embarrassment when I think about it.

While still on Risperidone I showed up at my friend's house with a delicious blueberry pound cake I had made. Everyone was shocked because this was not something I would do out of the blue. To this day we laugh about my "Manic Cake," as Line nicknamed it.

Risperidone made me feel almost euphoric at times, and I had energy I had never experienced. My family and friends noticed that I was acting in ways that were not typical of me. After doing some research on this drug I discovered that a rare side effect is "talking, feeling and acting with excitement and activity that cannot be controlled." The last day I took Risperidone, about five days after I started, was one of my scariest days since I was diagnosed with C-PTSD. I was on the phone with Lisa discussing my experience since starting this drug. At some point we talked about Jim being killed in the car accident, and my mouth began quivering and my whole body launched into violent shaking. I could not stop the movements. My legs kicked wildly, my feet stomped strongly on the floor, my arms flailed, my muscles stiffened, my eyes blinked uncontrollably, my lips smacked and puckered involuntarily. I was screaming, crying and speaking "in tongues" all at once. This bizarre behaviour went on for almost two hours. It was terrifying, and you can imagine how Lisa felt on the other end of the phone!

Not knowing what medical condition I had, I resorted to calling these episodes "tremors," although they were much more than a tremor. They were more like scenes from *The Exorcist*. My episodes looked and sounded like the exorcism on Regan (actress Linda Blair) in the film. They were bizarre!

I was seeing a psychologist, Dr. Donna McLennon, for Eye Movement Desensitization and Reprocessing (EMDR), a form of psychotherapy that has been known to effectively treat PTSD. I was hesitant but eager to try a new treatment. Dr. McLennon came highly recommended for her work with front-line personnel who witnessed trauma and some who have PTSD. I liked Donna, and it was obvious she had a solid understanding of trauma and EMDR. Although I realized that sometimes issues get worse before they get better in therapy, I became more and more anxious and overwhelmed as we went through my traumas, and I had to talk about them. I realized that EMDR was retraumatizing me. My nervous system was overloaded, and the seizures came on during EMDR, so I had to stop the therapy.

These incidents were the beginning of something no one—including my health-care professionals—were able to identify. I could be wrong, but I believe Risperidone was the culprit that started it. Within a week after the first incident the "tremors" became regular occurrences, lasting anywhere from forty-five minutes to five hours.

One such episode happened while I was waiting for a video conference appointment with my psychiatrist in Deer Lake. Lisa was attending the appointment with me, as I was quite unstable. As my total body tremors intensified so did my outbursts of screaming and loud babbling. Obviously, this attracted an audience, so a nurse in the building was called to my aid. She didn't know what to do and had no idea what was happening to me. Although I was terrified, I was adamant that I just wanted to go home. However, those who were attending to me felt it was their ethical responsibility to call 911. Within minutes a couple of paramedics entered the building. By this time, although I was fully aware of what was happening around me, I was incoherent. My daughter conferred with the paramedics and they decided to transport me to Western Memorial Regional Hospital in Corner Brook.

After an assessment in the emergency room, I was admitted to the psychiatric ward for observation. This four-hour episode ended with the help of Ativan which was administered intravenously. I slept well in a private room that night. Upon waking, a nurse directed me to the central area outside my room to pick up my breakfast tray. As I left the comfort of my room and saw the other patients, it hit me that I was on a psychiatric ward. My body started to tremble. The nurse assisted me back to my room and brought in my breakfast tray.

Dr. Du Toit, the psychiatrist on duty, and the attending nurse came to visit me shortly after breakfast. Seeing the psychiatrist walk in the room caused me to immediately experience stress in my body, which triggered the tremors. Dr. Du Toit asked me to explain what was happening. I gave him a brief description of my C-PTSD and of the most recent symptoms that landed me in the hospital. He continued to press me about my trauma. I found this extremely triggering and asked him to stop because he should know this was not appropriate.

"What do you want?" he asked.

"I just want to go home where I'm more comfortable," I quickly replied.

He agreed to discharge me and made contact with Dr. Walsh, my psychiatrist. Dr. Du Toit's notes from my Discharge Summary read: "Movements related to stress at home" and "Doesn't want to discuss nature of the trauma or when it occurred." Sadly, Dr. Du Toit and the other health-care professionals who were responsible for my care did not know what was wrong with me or how to treat it.

I had a second ambulance ride to Western Memorial Hospital a few weeks later. This time the tremors were severe and I was extremely vocal. The muscles around my neck and throat area began constricting and it became difficult to swallow. After over three hours and a different medication, the tremors slowed down and I returned home.

Following considerable inquiries that led to no answers, I took the matter into my own hands and began researching. My challenge was that I didn't know what to call my condition. Finally, I was able to "diagnose" myself with Psychogenic Non-Epileptic Seizures (PNES). When I took this turn for the worse, I couldn't have imagined that it was actually a blessing in disguise. I am grateful every day for my background, education and experience. Had I not been trained in the counselling field, I wouldn't have been able to diagnose myself and begin the healing process.

I've made it my mission to education others, especially mental-health professionals, about this condition. My psychiatrist, to my delight, took it upon himself to get training in PNES. My goal is to spread the word so others don't have to experience the frustration I did.

On April 6, 2018, while visiting my son in Labrador City, I was having a severe incident in the wee hours of the morning and reached out to the Mental Health Crisis Line. A man answered. I had difficulty speaking as I was having a seizure, and I was having severe flashbacks, panic, anxiety and was suicidal. Rather than helping me, the man on the line accused me of being drunk; he made me feel worthless and caused my symptoms to escalate. I was desperate, scared and couldn't get any help whatsoever from this man, so I hung up and called 911. This incident was traumatic for me.

When the dispatcher answered, I asked for Sam Coombs, a man I have known for many years and have complete trust in. Fortunately, he was there and was able to connect me to my counsellor. I talked to her on the phone until Sam and another paramedic arrived with the ambulance. They took me out of the apartment with a blanket over my head at my request, as I didn't want anyone to see me. I was ashamed and embarrassed because my seizures look bizarre. I was screaming, babbling incoherently and shaking uncontrollably. I was admitted to the hospital for five days.

I've had suicidal ideation on many occasions although I have never actually made a plan to follow through with my thoughts. I keep my medication in a plastic container in the bedroom closet. On the nights I was suicidal I gave Bill the container. This incident, however, was different; it was the closest I've ever come to taking my life. It's difficult to describe what overtook my mind. It was like nothing I had ever learned about in all the training I've received on suicide prevention and intervention. None of my suicidal clients described anything similar to what I experienced. When Sam put me on hold while he located my counsellor, I felt an intensely powerful force take control of my thoughts. The force moved into my head and was telling me to end my life. I couldn't escape it. Thankfully, my counsellor's soft voice on the phone brought me back to reality.

I frequently hear that suicide is a selfish act. If those who have taken their life experienced anything close to what I did that morning, I guarantee that the act is not selfish but entirely uncontrollable.

There are many triggers for me in Labrador City. On one of my return visits I decided to stay at a friend's apartment in the building where my EFAP office had been located. She was out of town so I had the place to myself, and it didn't occur to me that being in this building would be a trigger. I was alone very late at night. Suddenly, panic came rushing in and I started having a seizure. I was terrified and couldn't think straight. My brain was in a fog, and I knew I had to talk to someone or do something. I frantically called Hope Haven, a transition house for women and children, and spoke to the worker on call, Pat Pevie, whom I'd known for years. At first I felt awkward talking to Pat because she would see vulnerability she had never witnessed in me before. Within minutes any uneasiness I felt disappeared. Pat was understanding, caring and an excellent listener. As my brain was in a fog and I had difficulty concentrating, I'm not sure exactly how our conversation went. At some point, my friend Josephine's name came into the conversation. Pat and I agreed that she would contact Josephine and have her call me.

Pat woke Josephine up and she offered to come be with me. I quickly agreed and met her in the lobby of the apartment building. Josephine stayed with me after I had taken my medication until I was feeling sleepy. We chatted, I cried, she listened. She is an angel, one of the most compassionate and understanding women I know. I'm forever indebted to her for helping me through a very difficult night. I am blessed to have many friends in Labrador City who are only a phone call away and will go out of their way to help. Another call the following morning was to my friend, Cynt, who lives alone and was happy to have me stay with her for the remainder of my visit to Labrador City.

It would be so much easier to avoid places like Labrador City altogether. At an appointment with my counsellor we discussed exposure therapy, a proven method used to help break the pattern of avoidance and fear. As difficult as it would be, I knew I had to face my triggers in order to heal. And face them I did! I still have a few remaining but I'm well on the road to recovery, and I won't back down until all of them no longer have a hold on me. I want to be free.

On July 30, 2020, I had another severe incident while visiting my son in Labrador City. At 3:30 a.m. I began having a seizure, severe anxiety, racing thoughts, flashbacks and a fear that I would take my life. My service dog, Lily (I'll talk about her soon), stopped my seizure, but the other symptoms would not subside. This awful episode was triggered when I put Lily in her kennel, which I'd done dozens of times before. However, this time it brought my mind and body back to the numerous times I've been held against my will. Everything escalated to the point that I was afraid I was in serious trouble if I didn't get some help. I called the CHANNAL Warm Line in St. John's first and got the voicemail saying to leave a message and someone would call me back. A crisis line that sends a caller to voicemail? Astounding. There wasn't any indication when I could expect a call, and I needed someone immediately. I've since learned that the Warm Line is only staffed from 10 a.m. to midnight. Unfortunately, the voicemail didn't say the hours. I've given the CHANNAL feedback recommending that they put the hours of operation into their voicemail message.

I reluctantly called the Mental Health Crisis Line in St. John's. Because of my previous experience with the man on the crisis line, I was terrified that I would be triggered. When a man answered the phone, I knew I couldn't talk to him. It was difficult to concentrate, and my mind wandered back to that call in April 2018. My symptoms began to worsen, so I told the man I couldn't talk to him. He didn't question why, he just gave me some options. I then called the National Suicide Prevention Line and got a recording that said everyone was busy helping other people. I was left on hold listening to music for what seemed like an eternity. In the meantime, my symptoms were still escalating, and I was feeling more and more desperate.

I decided to call the emergency department at the hospital. I spoke to the nurse, explained my situation, asked if I could talk to her and she said I could. However, our conversation was completely one-sided. At one point I asked if she was still there because she was silent. This didn't feel comfortable and wasn't helping me. I asked her a couple questions and soon realized that she had no experience whatsoever in counselling. I'm not knocking her for this—taking my crisis call was not her job, after all—but she didn't know where to direct me.

Thankfully, I am a resourceful person whose career path lead me to leave no stone unturned until I found the help others needed. This has served me well. I instinctively knew I needed to talk to someone to alleviate my symptoms. I didn't want to call family or friends in the wee hours of the morning. There are many people who would have gladly taken my call, but I didn't want to wake anyone. There was only one more place in Labrador City that I could call. I searched the number for Hope Haven, and my angel was surely watching out for me.

Two hours after the episode began I hung up the phone from talking to a counsellor at Hope Haven. I could finally think clearly and was not having flashbacks from some of my many traumas, particularly the trauma when I was held against my will. I wasn't having a seizure thanks to Lily. My anxiety had disappeared, and I was no longer afraid I would commit suicide. The counsellor at Hope Haven, who talked to me for what must have been close to an hour, was amazingly compassionate and understanding. I told her I was going to write about this experience but, the modest woman she is, said I shouldn't use her name. I send my gratitude to the Hope Haven counsellor; she just may have saved my life.

This incident finally gave me the courage to pursue my concerns with the service provided by the provincial Mental Health Crisis Line. I wrote letters to a number of different officials outlining the events which occurred and recommended actions I felt could improve the service. The response I received wasn't to my satisfaction, but I'm hoping that bringing the matter to their attention will, in some small way, make a difference. I have satisfaction in knowing that I tried.

Just prior to the start of my PNES I decided to try medical cannabis for my mental illness. It was 2016 and using cannabis was illegal unless you had a prescription. My psychiatrist and family doctor were supportive of me trying it but were unable to prescribe it. Coincidentally, CBC aired a story about the opening of a cannabinoid clinic when I was searching. I booked an appointment with their psychiatrist, hoping he would prescribe cannabis for my mental illness. As requested, my doctor mailed a complete medical file to the clinic. I was also required to complete a number of pre-visit questionnaires (i.e., CAGE, Medical Cannabis Initial Assessment), which were emailed to me and returned to the clinic.

Although my appointment was scheduled for 11, the psychiatrist didn't call me until around 11:25. He advised that the appointment was for one hour and this included the time he spent to review my file. He told me he rarely prescribes cannabis for his patients. I then spent approximately ten minutes in his office. I described my medical condition to him—anxiety, memory issues, inability to concentrate, previous therapies.

"You must be a really good actress because you aren't showing any of these symptoms," he said.

"Yes I am," I responded. "I've spent my whole life acting."

I thought he was being sincere, however, as I've had time to reflect on this comment, I realize his tone of voice and body language were intended to degrade me. He asked me to describe my medical condition again.

"I have Complex PTSD," I said.

"What is that and when did it start?" he asked.

"Are you asking because you don't know what the illness is or do you want me to describe what I believe the illness to be?"

He asked me how the illness affected my life, so I explained that it began at birth with the death of my identical twin sister. As I began to explain that it controls my life, I could no longer "act" because of the stress I felt, and my body went into a seizure. Before the appointment began, I asked the doctor if he was aware of my seizures, and I had phoned the clinic to advise them that it was quite possible that I could have one during my appointment, as they come on when I am under stress. He said, in quite a sarcastic tone, that there was a big note on the file regarding it. This psychiatrist showed no concern whatsoever for my distress. He opened the office door and asked me to leave. I told him I wanted to ask him some questions and asked him to please close the door for privacy.

"I won't talk to you while you're shaking," he said.

"Do you think I can stop?"

He told me it was time for my husband to come get me. The doctor stated that he had his mind made up before he saw me and that he would not prescribe cannabis as I was actively in my illness. He wasn't there to entertain me, he said, so I should stop wasting his time. I told him he was rude and had no empathy or sympathy. By this time, Bill, who watched the incident unfold, was helping me leave the office. As the doctor closed the door I realized that the staff and patients in the waiting area were privy to this entire exchange; I was humiliated.

When I obtained a copy of the psychiatrist's report which was sent to my family doctor, it stated that he did not believe I have seizures but that the shaking is "histrionic in nature." I took great offence to this accusation; attention seeking is the last thing a person who suffers from PNES wants. He went on to assess me as a "personality disordered individual, with significant dependent traits." It took a couple of long sessions with Dr. Walsh, my psychiatrist, to diagnose my C-PTSD, so how could this man properly make a diagnosis in a ten-minute appointment? Why would he write such degrading information to my family doctor, a man whom I see on a regular basis?

I was required to give a urine sample at the clinic, and it tested positive for opiates. In his report to my family doctor, the psychiatrist stated that this was "of interest to me as none of the medication listed, despite the lengthy list, includes opiates." Again, this illustrates his attempt to degrade me, essentially saying that I was using opiates. I asked my pharmacist to research my medication, and he discovered the antidepressant Pristiq, which I take daily, may interfere with urine detection of phencyclidine, showing a false-positive. This man, an educated psychiatrist, should have known this information.

Although it took two years and numerous attempts, I wrote a complaint letter to The College of Physicians and Surgeons of Newfoundland and Labrador. Each attempt resulted in severe anxiety and seizures, but I refused to give up. The committee reviewing my complaint called the psychiatrist to task regarding how he treated me. He acknowledged that he "may have been somewhat abrupt and could have taken extra time to help ground [Ms. Samson] prior to ending the session." He also wrote me a letter of apology which is not worth the paper it's written on; it's fake. However, I am satisfied that I stood up for myself, and I hope that my exposure of his unprofessional behaviour will help him remember to treat other patients with the respect they deserve.

TRE®

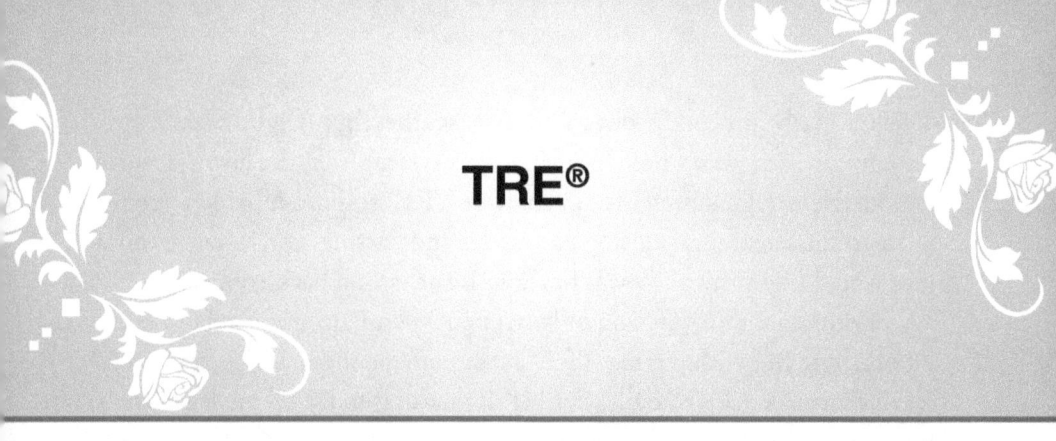

On the drive home from the cannabinoid clinic, I had an epiphany. I was having a seizure while rehashing the events at the clinic with Bill. Suddenly, I came to the realization that the seizures were mimicking the TRE® that I had learned a number of years prior, particularly the trembling. In this moment of clarity I wondered if TRE® would help my seizures.

After suffering with C-PTSD and now PNES, I was desperate. Something inside me was saying I needed to give TRE® a shot, so my desperation transformed into countless hours of TRE® in the loft over our garage—just me and the blue gym mat Damian gave me. I am forever grateful for it. I kept notes about my long and intense 1.5- to 2.5-hour TRE® sessions. My body rocked and shook violently, and I screamed so loud that my throat was sore. I cried, babbled and uttered primitive sounds. Some of the very long sessions were extremely intense, and we were thankful that we lived in a secluded area where my vicious screams that accompanied the release of my trauma couldn't be heard by others. I'm sure they would have resulted in a 911 call. There was a time in my life that this intensity would have scared me. However, I was blessed to be in a position where I was far enough along in my healing that I could "let go" and allow my body to do what it needed to heal. I felt safe and looked forward to my daily retreat to the loft.

After a month of daily TRE®, I had a session which left me completely overwhelmed and at a loss for words. It felt as though a "guiding force" did acupressure and then guided my hand to a lump in my breast (which was benign). Again, I started researching and learned that this phenomenon is known as myofascial release.

Gradually my body began to release the fight/flight/freeze/fawn responses which were stored in my nervous system from the horrific abuse I endured throughout my life. There were TRE® sessions in which I could relate to the screaming, tensing of muscles and cursing, and it was in those moments I knew my body was healing. I was taking back control.

Seizures are rare now and only happen when I am triggered or have a lot of stress. But with regular TRE® I can manage them. Lily is trained to remind me to do TRE® daily. For her, it's natural to lay on my legs, being bounced around, while the trauma shakes out of my body. Although I am not cured from C-PTSD or PNES, I am on the road to recovery.

Medical Cannabis

In my search to find someone to prescribe medical cannabis I found Marijuana for Trauma, an organization staffed by volunteers who set up a Skype appointment with a doctor. This doctor asked a few questions and, without hesitation, prescribed medical cannabis for me. I had no idea it could be so easy.

The challenge came when I began using cannabis, as I was not given instructions regarding how much to take. When my order arrived, I contacted a veteran who got PTSD when he was in the military to ask his advice about dosage. He was a great guy to talk to, had a good understanding of mental illness and had been using cannabis to help with his condition for a long time. As he wasn't trained to give expert advice, he could only offer me his understanding of how the product worked for him. I carefully wrote down the dosage he used, as it was the only guidelines I had to follow at the time. Without an understanding of CBD and TCH I decided to use the same dosage as he was using. This is where it gets interesting.

Melv delivered my parcel, and I was eager to get started. He and Bill were getting ready to do some work on our water supply. As I laid the syringes and cannabis bottles on the table I felt a nervous excitement. I was hopeful that this new treatment would provide more relief from my symptoms of C-PTSD. Checking the notes I had made when I consulted with the veteran, I carefully measured the cannabis oil according to his experience. As I pushed the oil from the syringe into my mouth I shuddered at the taste—bitter, earthy and kind of like how oil smells. I quickly washed the taste away with a glass of water.

I cautiously went about my daily routine, anxiously awaiting to feel the effect of my new drug. I didn't know what to expect. Suddenly I realized I was on the stairway landing beside the porch, confused and huddled in the corner. Bill appeared beside me, looking bewildered.

"Deb, what are you doing?"

"I don't know how to get out of here," I said.

He couldn't comprehend what was wrong with me, so I had to repeat myself several times before it registered. He patiently escorted me through the porch and into the living room. I was wandering aimlessly around the house and stepped into the kitchen where Bill was preparing his lunch. I stood in one spot while Bill manoeuvred around me.

"What are you doing?" he asked again.

"I don't know how to get out of here," I said again.

I laugh to myself as I recall Bill's words: "Just walk somewhere else." From Bill's perspective this seemed simple, but I was under the influence of the TCH in my cannabis, so it was challenging. Having used illicit drugs in my teens, I knew I was stoned. Bill has never been stoned in his life, so he had difficulty comprehending my state of mind and was concerned for my safety. Although he was preparing to work on the water supply, I asked him not to leave as I was scared.

Line came to the rescue. It was a glorious summer day, so we sat on the patio, enjoying the warm sunshine, gentle breeze and breathtaking view of the ocean. The paranoia and fear I was experiencing had turned into a jovial mood. I was relaxed and had no inhibition whatsoever. I could not stop talking and changed topics in mid-sentence. I didn't give Line a chance to speak. I would look at the smirk on her face and laughingly tell her to "fuck off." Line, like Bill, has no understanding of what it's like to be stoned. She seemed quite amused by my giggly, chatty behaviour. She thought it was hilarious.

As the day passed, the effects of my cannabis high gradually subsided. I realized I would need to do much research before attempting another dose. When I placed my cannabis order I asked for one to help me sleep. It had a high THC content, and I was unaware that I have a very low tolerance to THC. I do, however, need to use a small amount with my CBD in order to sleep well. Not knowing the difference, this time I ordered cannabis with too much THC.

I'm a night owl who is generally on a 3 a.m. to 11 a.m. schedule. Bill usually goes to bed around ten o'clock, so when I decided to try the first dose of night-time cannabis, Bill was fast asleep. I reluctantly measured the oil into a syringe, squirted it in my mouth and washed it down with water. I waited for an hour and, not feeling any effects, I felt safe to go to bed. My head was barely laid on the pillow when I realized I was stoned. The white noise machine is always on when I sleep, but I heard a soft male voice repeating different phrases such as "The wheel is turning," "Go get the bottle," etc. I was having audio hallucinations. I listened to the words that made no sense and tried, unsuccessfully, to block them out. When I got high as a teenager I had vivid hallucinations, but this was a whole different experience.

Realizing that I would not get to sleep, I decided to get up. Upon entering the bathroom, which is just around the corner from the bedroom, my audio hallucinations were replaced by visual ones. When I looked at the grain in the flooring I saw unfamiliar faces rising up. Bill was fast asleep, and I felt somewhat uneasy, not knowing what to expect. As I sat on the stool at the kitchen peninsula I knew I needed to talk to someone who had an understanding of cannabis. Lisa's caring words entered my thoughts: "Mom, call me anytime you need me; I don't care what time it is."

I speed dialled Lisa's number and was relieved to hear her reassuring voice. While I was telling her about the effects from the cannabis, I shouted, "I see the face of Jesus coming out of the kitchen floor!" We laughed uncontrollably.

"I don't think there are many mothers who could call their daughter and have a conversation like this!" she said with a laugh.

She reassured me that what I was experiencing was normal and that she was there for me. Lisa often tells this story when she is advocating for cannabis use to help others with medical issues. It's a funny memory that has been retold many times.

Bill says he sleeps with one eye open because he never knows what to expect from me in the night-time, so all of this commotion woke him. I finished my conversation with Lisa while Bill listened on trying to understand what was happening. As I hung up the phone and turned to look at Bill, his face became part of my next hallucination. It was morphing, in slow motion, into a cartoon type character. I found it funny, but Bill didn't seem to be amused; he just wanted me to go to bed. I explained that I was stoned and didn't think I could go to sleep. He insisted that I give it a try so, to give him the benefit of the doubt, I went back to bed. Nothing had changed, I was still hallucinating.

Bill was concerned for my well-being and wanted to stay up with me, but I assured him I would call if I needed to. I was confident I could ride this out, and I did.

Before proceeding further with my trial of medical cannabis I poured over vast amounts of information on the internet. I made inquiries with my supplier and eventually found what worked for me. Using medical cannabis was a game changer for me; it helped to reduce the amount of prescription medication I had been consuming, and it has given me an overall sense of well-being. I now use only CBD oil in the daytime. My night-time cannabis consists of half CBD and half TCH and has been very helpful for my insomnia. There was much trial and error, but I'm happy I stuck with it until I found the right dosage for me.

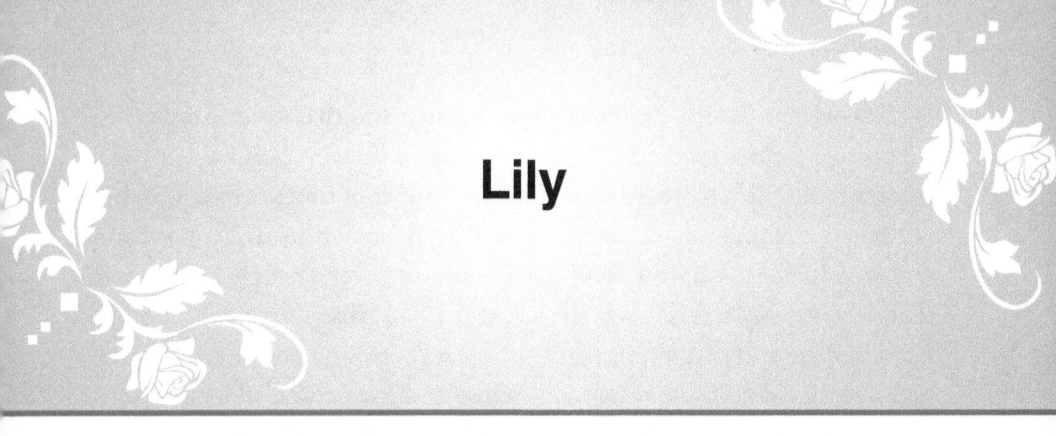

Lily

I decided to get a psychiatric service dog. After much consultation with professionals I felt the best route to expedite the process was to buy a dog and train it myself. Enter my Havanese service dog, Lily. We call Lily our magic little pill because this twelve-pound miracle stops my seizures.

I decided to get a Havanese because they are easy to train and low maintenance. After doing my homework, I made contact with Paradise Kennel in New Brunswick and chose my tiny black and white fluffy ball of love. From the moment I saw her picture I was in love. That love and bond grew stronger from the moment I held her in my arms at the airport.

It was quite by accident that we discovered Lily can stop my seizures. Not long after getting Lily, Bill put her in my lap while I was having a seizure and it immediately stopped. We looked at each other in awe. Was this a coincidence? It wasn't long before there was another opportunity to test Lily's "magic," so Bill put her in my lap when my seizure started and, again, the seizure stopped. We were amazed!

We needed to test our theory. While I was having a seizure, Bill put Line's dog, Ginger, in my lap, but the seizure continued. On another occasion, while visiting my son, Bill put his cat, Ninj, in my lap; again, the seizure continued. Both Ginger and Ninj are cuddly, loving animals whom I have a bond with, so we proved our Lily theory.

Thus, Lily became my service dog. We quickly built a bond, and she is my constant companion. She travels with me, accompanies me to the doctor, visits with friends, goes shopping and gets quite upset if there is a rare occasion when I leave the house without her. She is a blessing in my time of need. The love and compassion I feel from Lily has developed into a relationship of devotion which I never could have imagined. We are inseparable.

Having a service dog has been mostly positive, and people are supportive for the most part. On one occasion, however, Bill and I went to a restaurant where we had taken Lily a number of times before. On this particular evening one of the owners, who is known to us, stopped me and said I couldn't have Lily in her restaurant. Even though I explained that Lily was my service dog, she asked if I had papers for her. I told her I did but she still wouldn't permit us to eat there. She said she had never had a service dog in the restaurant before and she needed to look into it. A business owner has a responsibility to know the regulations regarding access for persons with disabilities who have service dogs. She could have taken a minute to look it up online. However, she was adamant that we were not allowed to eat at her restaurant if Lily was with us.

I took this matter to social media in an effort to educate the public, business owners in particular, about service dogs. The local media heard of my story and asked for an interview. CBC aired the story and it drew quite a bit of attention. I hope the restaurant owner and others have gained a better understanding of the regulations for service dogs in Newfoundland and Labrador as a result of my unfortunate experience.

I work with an amazing trainer who is assisting me with Lily's training. It's hard work, but well worth the effort.

Even before Lily was born I knew I wanted a female dog, and I was going to name her Lily. My Aunt Lily, who passed away a few years ago, was a woman who had a positive influence on my life. Saying "Lily" each time I call my little dog evokes a feeling of pleasure and brings a smile to my face.

We Must Do Better for the Children

My calling to help people has shifted, and I have a new, slightly different mission. I now aim to educate others through my story instead of my work. Out of suffering comes clarity and purpose.

I hope that parents and other adults will educate themselves about the effects of adverse childhood experiences. By telling my story of trauma, I believe good will come from it and others will avert a diagnosis of C-PTSD and/or PNES. These illnesses are entirely preventable! The general public needs to know and understand how experiences such as abuse, violence and dysfunction can affect brain development and the nervous system, which can lead to various problems such as mental illness, addiction, eating disorders and other chronic diseases. Just as we tell parents to ensure their child wears a helmet when riding their bike, we need to tell parents to prevent their child from being traumatized. We can avoid a public health crisis through education.

I have witnessed children taken into the "system" out of concern for their well-being only to be placed back into the same environment. These children were traumatized. I've watched, with sadness, as they've grown into teenagers who cut themselves, develop eating disorders, experience anxiety, addictions and various other issues all as a result of their trauma. Common sense tells us that not every trauma can be averted. Witnessing an accident, for example, is usually unavoidable. When trauma occurs, children often need professional intervention. When trauma can be prevented, we have a responsibility as a society to protect our vulnerable children. Public health officials spring into action with awareness campaigns, as they should, around such things as injuries to children on trampolines, so they should take the same action when it comes to childhood trauma!

Many health professionals who are responsible for our children's well-being are not properly trained in the area of childhood trauma and aren't given the appropriate tools and authority to intervene and take the necessary action to protect our children. I am appalled that our antiquated "system" is failing children in the 2020s the same way it failed me in the 1970s. It's fifty years later, we have to do better!

Life Today

I am sixty-two years old. On January 1, 2021, I officially retired from my job with thirty years of service. I posted an announcement on Facebook (with my employer's name eliminated to protect their identity) when I retired. I wanted people to know what happened to me and that I didn't get "the boot" (as some had assumed) when the EFAP office was closed. It was an opportunity to thank my employer and the many individuals who helped me fulfil my dream and calling of helping others.

Now I am finally carrying out one of the major items on my bucket list. For as long as I can remember I've wanted to write a book about my life. Many others have encouraged and inspired me, and I've made several attempts, but I had to discard them because I wasn't ready. In the early years it was because I couldn't get my writing to "flow," but recently triggering events thwarted my writing. As I gaze at the words I've written, I feel many emotions: gratitude for the people who have supported and encouraged me along the way, relief that I've finally gotten it out of my head and on paper, joy that my experiences will help others, and thankfulness that I survived to tell my story. I have chosen to speak my truth, as painful as it has been. I've faced many of my triggers while writing my story, and writing about them has been incredibly therapeutic.

I have concerns about how the people who have hurt me will react to my disclosure. I do not want to cause them pain. I'm fearful that their reactions may set me back in my healing because stress and anxiety are my enemies. After discussing this with my daughter, she reminded me of a quote by Anne Lamott: "You own everything that happened to you. Tell your stories. If people wanted you to write warmly about them, they should've behaved better."

I wanted to believe there would be no more trauma but life often has things in store which could never be anticipated. As I sit here, after having a seizure, I am grateful for my service dog, Lily, who stopped it.

The phone call I received today from David will be forever etched in my mind. He was very angry that I've written my story, used derogatory language and called me a "fucking bitch" (the same language used by his step-daughter when she called me the previous day).

I am still in shock and disbelief as I recall the words that came out of his mouth.

"I want to strangle you."

"When you do that book launch in Eastport I will be there and you will be sorry."

"I will show up in your driveway and give you a dammed good fright."

"I'm going to kill you. I'm going to shoot you".

The RCMP have a file on this incident. They have been in contact with David.

As difficult as this is, I will not allow threats, even death threats, to stop me. I will tell my truth and I will help others in the process!

Bill has been my constant support; he could write a book, I'm sure. It hasn't been easy for him. He says that he no longer has to sleep with one eye open. Every night when I "tuck him in," he says, "You know where I am if you need me." He never forgets those words; they remind me that, with his unwavering love and support, I'll be okay.

Riding the roller coaster of mental illness has not only been difficult for me. My family and friends have watched on, often feeling helpless. Although they may not have realized it, just being with me or validating my feelings was all I needed from them. Together we have navigated the waters of C-PTSD and PNES. We've learned together, cried and laughed, but, most importantly, we've endured.

My son coined the term "fish flop" when I began having seizures. When he phones me and hears a quiver in my voice he asks, "Mom, are you doing the fish flop again?" Being able to joke and laugh about my mental illnesses has brought much needed relief to a serious matter.

The first time Melv rounded the corner into the kitchen and saw me having a seizure, he thought I was pretending to dance and was about to engage with me in a good ole Newfie jig. We have laughed about this moment many times.

My daughter has been my constant "go to" about my writing. She is an excellent writer and has provided valuable coaching along the way. She knows my story intimately. At one point I asked her to promise that if I died before my book was finished, she would finish it for me; she agreed.

A few years ago I began practicing gratitude. A friend on Facebook posted a challenge to write one thing I was grateful for each day for thirty days. This became an almost two-year journey of being thankful for the many blessings in my life each and every day. Practicing gratitude changed my life. Although I don't write it on paper every day, I constantly look for the good things in my life. As I write, I take a moment to gaze out the window, looking at the calmness of the ocean, the brightness of the sun on a cloudless day, the stillness of the trees, water dripping off the roof as the snow melts away. I savour the beauty around me and soak up the feeling of gratitude for all that I am blessed with. Life is good.

Soon after moving to Fox Point, Line introduced me to a fun hobby. We spend a lot of time walking on the beaches, and one time she stopped to pick up something, and that is when I learned about sea glass. Many years ago it was acceptable for residents to throw their garbage in the ocean, so there was a lot of glass floating around. Over time, the ocean has worn it down to beautiful sea glass pieces. Now, in addition to knitting, quilting and crocheting I create sea glass art. It takes a considerable amount of time, as I have to collect, sort and wash the glass before I produce my art. I've covered old house windows with beautiful creations such as inukshuks, butterflies, horses, birds, frogs, cats and dogs just to name a few. I also put my sea glass art on various size pictures. I make sea glass sun catchers, coasters and signs. Bill makes rustic birch end tables for Line and I to put our sea glass creations on. I'm so very grateful to have found this hobby. It is tremendously therapeutic.

Bill just celebrated his sixty-fifth birthday. We had a barbeque at our home with family and friends. At one point there were fourteen people in our home, including a crying baby and lots of conversations. We ended off the evening with a couple of card games with Line and Melv. There was a time not so long ago that this amount of stimulation would have been awfully difficult for me and even would have caused a seizure. Not this time; the evening was so very enjoyable. There was no brain fog or anxiety, and I was able to concentrate while we played cards. I know my brain is healing; it takes time and hard work, but it is possible.

Yes, my "biological" family has disowned me, but… I now have a "chosen" family. When Rev. Florence Sanna asked, "Debbie, if you could have chosen your parents, would you have chosen Jim and Ruby?" she set me on a path that brought more true love into my life than I ever could have imagined. Family is not defined by a bloodline but by those people in your circle who are your lifeline. I am grateful to have a lifeline no matter where I go.

www.ingramcontent.com/pod-product-compliance
Lightning Source LLC
LaVergne TN
LVHW041639060526
838200LV00040B/1639